The Wandering Womb

The Wandering Womb

A Cultural History of Outrageous Beliefs About Women

Lana Thompson

Foreword by Vern L. Bullough

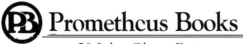

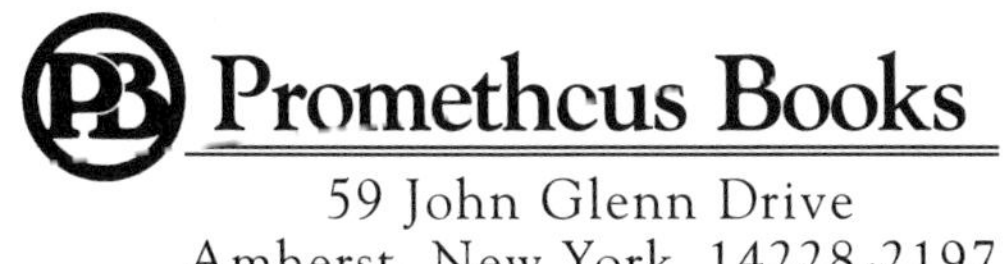

59 John Glenn Drive
Amherst, New York 14228-2197

To Jenny and Hannah

Published 1999 by Prometheus Books

02 01 00 99 5 4 3 2 1

Library of Congress Cataloging-in-Publication Data

Thompson, Lana.
The wandering womb : a cultural history of outrageous beliefs about women / by Lana Thompson ; foreword by Vern L. Bullough.
p. cm.
Includes index.
ISBN 1–57392–264–1 (alk. paper)
1. Women—Folklore. 2. Women—Physiology. 3. Body, Human—Folklore. 4. Sex—Folklore. 5. Sex—Mythology. I. Title.
GR470.T53 1999
398′.3′082—dc21 98–51678
CIP

Printed in the United States of America on acid-free paper

Contents

Acknowledgments

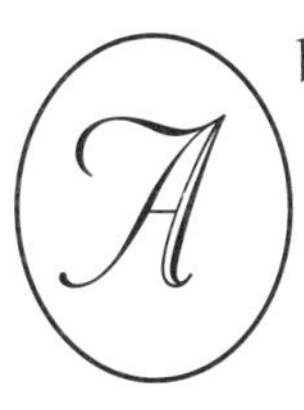

A book would not be complete without some personal history of its construction. The author was both encouraged and (like the uterus) suffered many outrageous comments.

Thank you to:

David Washburn—who encouraged me to write, though it wasn't until I gained access to tool technology (in the form of a computer) that I could practice.

Ann Peyton—who let me take her creative-writing class. She doled out kindness and patience as well as constructive criticism in measures that never hurt . . . not one bit. I admire her for her tact when I look at my early papers.

Ronald Shellow—who liked my letters.

Eleanor Schuster—who allowed me to participate in her "Women, Witches, and Healing" and "Women's Health Issues" seminars.

Usha Sudhakar—who worked diligently to find me all the books I needed for interlibrary loan, as well as Ken Frankel and Bill Armstrong, who helped me research the old requests when I needed to reorder; and Carlos Nelson, university librarian, collection development, and Rita Pellen, associate director for libraries, women's studies librarian, in the reference department, whose knowledge and experience was awesome (for lack of a better word). Carlos and Rita both helped me during panic attacks when I needed a journal over the weekend.

Susan L. Brown—who let me take her "Gender and Nonwestern Culture" class, offered to read my first draft, and typed out six pages of comments over one weekend. Dr. Brown is the only person who volunteered to read my manuscript and actually did.

Dee Ray—who took the time to let me know she cared even after her own life was pummeled by traumatic events.

Julie Pavlon—Assistant Director of Women's Studies, who encouraged me to pursue my goals.

David Graves—the radiologist who provided his personal collection of *Journals of the American Medical Association* to me.

Betsy Cox—who saved the journals when I didn't come to pick them up.

Richard Cavanagh—who answered questions about nomenclature no matter how busy he was.

Len Washburn—whose enthusiasm and interest, as well as comfort and care, helped me through the entire journey.

Leon Blostein—who believed enough in the value of knowledge to show me a dog's uterus despite the objections of my parents and other adults who thought it "inappropriate." Leon surrendered four of his precious veterinary books, important to my preliminary research for this book.

Vern Bullough—who provided me with invaluable comments and opinions on my draft.

The women at AAUW—who were interested enough in my original paper to ask me to read it.

Leo Waldstein and Vaslav Nijinsky—my cats, who were

always happy to see me, even when I was working at the computer keyboard. Mr. Waldstein died on September 22, 1998.

Susan Waide—who provided art that I could never have obtained on my own.

Eric Luft—who helped with last-minute images, personally tracking the progress.

Helen Bannan—the first director of women's studies, who left too soon to share the rewards.

Dr. A. M. Luyendijk-Elshout—who lived at the University during World War II and shared her personal history as well as the history of the original Leiden operating theater and books in the medical library with me.

And lastly, to the memory of Otto Bettmann, the "picture man" and creator of the Bettmann Archive. Otto discouraged me from the entire project, saying it had far too many pictures and not enough sex. He then bragged incessantly about my "you-ter-us" book in his delightful German accent. Otto died May 1, 1998, at the age of 94.

Foreword

BY VERN L. BULLOUGH

Throughout much of history, and even to some extent today, definitions about women's place and role in society and in the family have been made by men. It is the attempt of women to define for themselves what they can and should be and do that is the cornerstone of modern feminism. Women—men have historically felt—were somehow radically different from themselves. They not only lacked a penis (which somehow made them inferior), but they also gave birth through a rather mysterious process that took place in their bodies. The female power to give birth was both worshiped by men and used as a justification to keep them under control. Males—who often stood in awe of the whole process of pregnancy—also tried to explain it, and some of the explanations made by men are the subject of this book.

Many ancient writers believed that the womb or uterus had a life of its own, and a *hystera* (the Greek term) wanted and needed to be filled (i.e., pregnant). In fact, if a woman was not regularly pregnant, she would suffer from *hysteria,* a catch-all category for somatic symptoms stimulating almost any kind of physical disease or mental condition. Hysteria was therefore something that only females suffered from—not males, who were of course vastly superior in all respects. To make matters worse, women not only gave birth, they also menstruated, another mysterious process that was not fully explained until the third decade of this century.

Physicians, in general, knew little about women, and so much of their care throughout Western history fell to the midwife. Unfortunately, midwives were not particularly well-educated (women as a whole were not), and so in cases of crisis pregnancy or a general family illness, physicians or surgeons could then intervene. Due to various moral proscriptions, however, physicians were not permitted to examine women as thoroughly as they could their male patients. This began to change with the appearance of male midwives, the forerunner of modern obstetricians, who gained a foothold in the birthing industry through the invention of the forceps in the seventeenth century, an instrument which made difficult births somewhat easier. The real turning point, however, was the development of anesthesia in the last half of the nineteenth century, since control of anesthesia was in the hands of the physician. The result was the medicalization of child birth and, in countries like the United States, the elimination of midwifery as a profession. Once medicine became dominant and the birthing process moved into the hospitals, the midwives found themselves being pushed out since they could not get hospital appointments.

Still, medical students were taught very little about female anatomy or the problems of delivery until the twentieth century. Indeed, even as late as the last half of the nineteenth century, a professor at the University of Buffalo who had his students examine a pregnant woman came in for public condemnation. By the twentieth century, the obstetrician had become dominant and what some would call the Age of Heroic Obstetrics developed. Some prominent physicians even regarded pregnancy as a pathological condition that required all kinds of intervention. The nursing of babies was discouraged by most obstetricians, and women who did so were often looked down upon until the 1950s.

In today's world, we can look back in wonder at many of the ideas concerning women in the past, and Lana Thompson, in this illustrated and light-hearted (but scholarly) overview, does just that. In the process, she helps us to understand why feminism as a movement was so important, and how scientific assumptions have often been shaped by social prejudices that are very difficult to overcome.

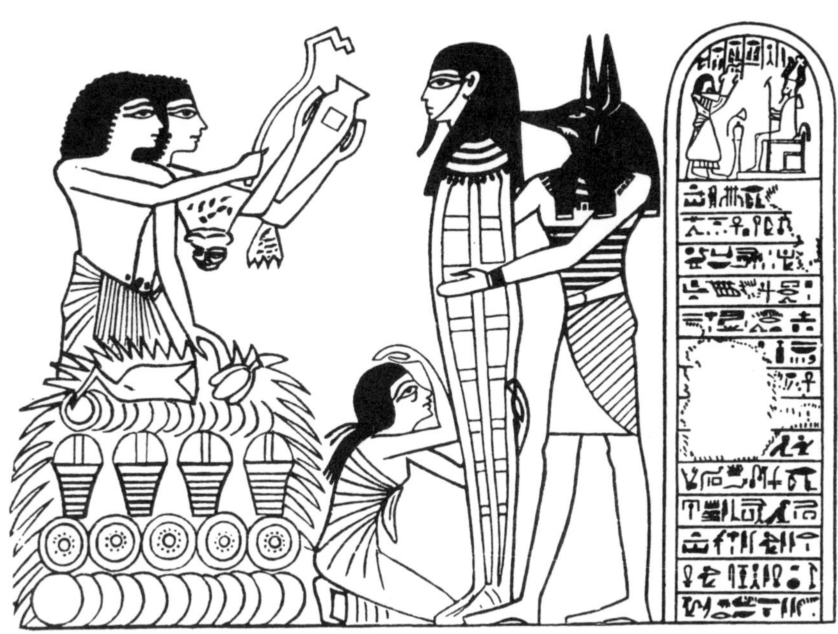

The belief in a womb that wanders can be traced to Egyptian antiquity.

Introduction

The uterus of the woman on the bed contracted according to its cellular intelligence. Without command the vertical muscles squeezed downward. The woman moaned. The sound rose slowly in the thick bed. The downward rippling of the vertical muscles jammed to a halt against the horizontal muscles at the bag's narrow neck. The uterus was wide, its neck was narrow, the horizontal muscles strove outward now to make the circle wider. At this time, in the timelessness of the cell, the contractions of the uterus were occurring at three-minute intervals. . . . When the first tentative contractions splayed in her pelvis, the will of the uterus barely fingered the threshold of pain.

—*The Cry and the Covenant,* Morton Thompson

Any book that attempts, however briefly, to chronicle the history of outrageous beliefs about women must first at least touch on the question of why those beliefs came into being. How did we develop the social codes that govern the relations between women and men? Creation myths, those metaphoric or symbolic stories that explain how people account for their existence, codify their social relationships, and establish order, are found

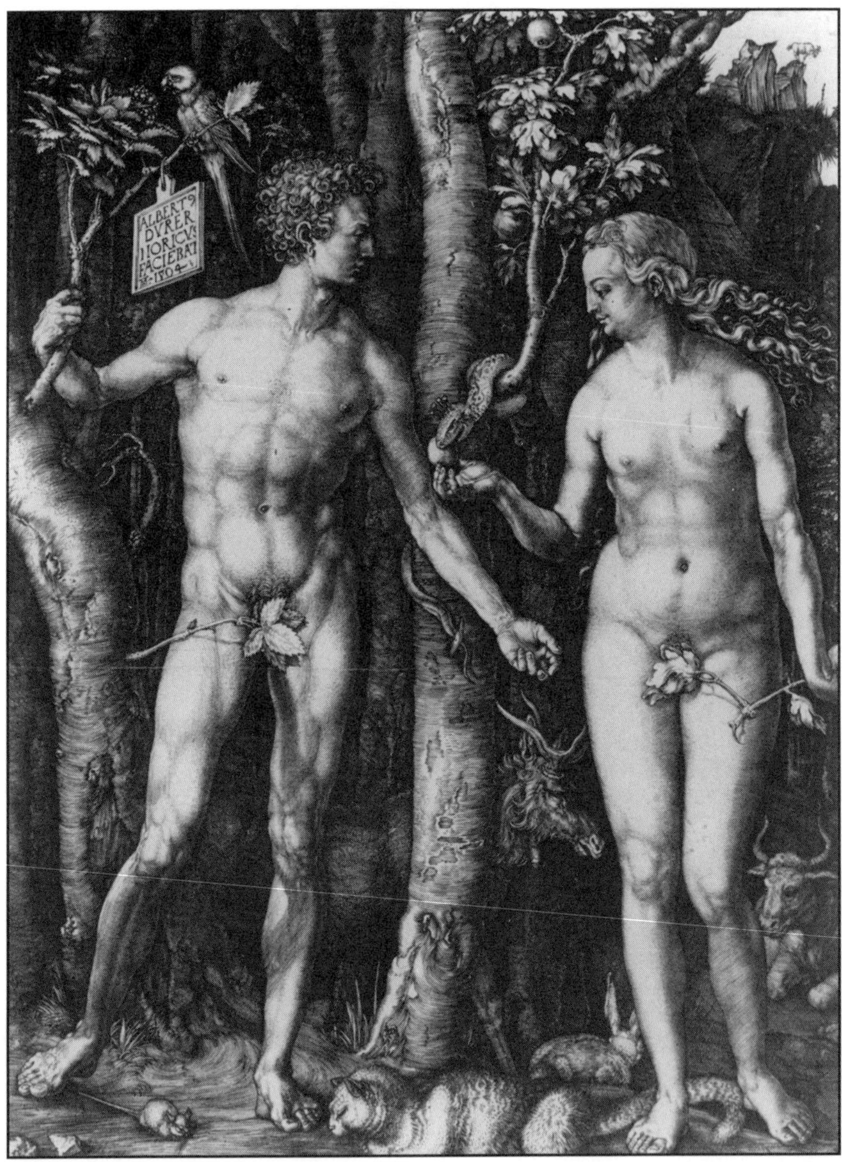

Albrecht Dürer (1471–1528). *Adam and Eve.* Engraving. Location not indicated. Courtesy: FOTO Marburg/Art Resource, New York.

***Figure 1.* The Primal Pair in the Garden of Eden.** Our culture's perception of women is based on the Judeo-Christian creation myth, which teaches that woman is not only inferior to man in body and mind, but that she is the source of all his frustrations and temptations. To dispel such notions, one must do more than count ribs.

In this engraving by Albrecht Dürer, Eve is shown tempting Adam with fruit from the tree of knowledge. According to the creation myth, this fruit was forbidden because it would make mortals like gods. Although Adam chose to partake, Eve was blamed for his behavior. As a result of her "seduction," the two were driven from paradise by an angry God.

The blame assigned to Eve for tempting Adam with forbidden fruit lies at the core of many assumptions about women's psychological nature. Medical decisions, especially ones related to childbirth, reproduction, and sexuality, have been shaded by this prejudice throughout the ages. Indeed, when anesthetics were first introduced in medicine, the biblical proscription "All women must bring forth children in sorrow" was one reason used to deny them to women in labor.

---

in every culture. They provide us with important clues about the people who wrote or told them.

Many cultures pattern their gender relationships on a social structure that is attributed in turn to their particular supernatural hierarchy of human and non-human deities.[1] In Western cultures, the Bible serves as the model for that structure. It tells the story of a male God who created a male and female primal pair in rank order: first Adam, later Eve. The couple was given instructions about their small world, with a peculiar restriction. They were not to eat the fruit of a certain tree, the tree of the knowledge of good and evil. If they did, their Creator told them, they would "surely die." And so Adam and Eve lived in harmony with this injunction until a snake convinced Eve that she would surely *not* die if she ate of the forbidden tree. So Eve "saw that the tree was good for food, and that it was pleasant to the eyes, and a tree to be desired to make one wise, [and] she took the fruit thereof, and did eat, and gave also unto her husband with her."[2] But the male God soon learned that the couple knew about nakedness (which was somehow connected to the concept of good and evil) and inquired, "Who told thee that thou wast naked?" Adam replied, "The woman whom thou gavest to be with me, she gave me of the

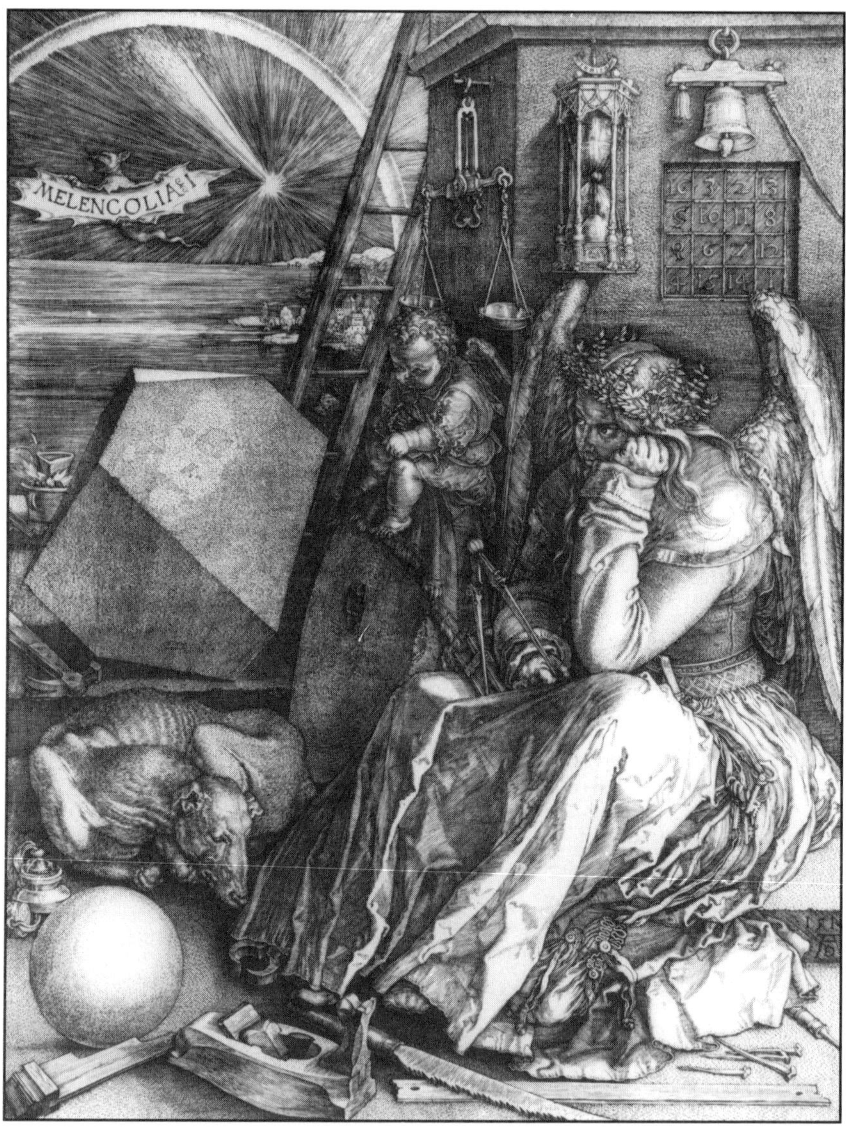

Albrecht Dürer (1471–1528). *Melencolia I,* 1514. Location not indicated. Courtesy: FOTO Marburg/Art Resource, New York.

***Figure 2.* The Humoral Theory.** During the time of Hippocrates, the humoral theory explained the etiology of disease. The body, like the universe, was thought to be composed of four elements: earth, air, water, and fire. Galen used these terms to characterize personality, associating each one to a particular temperament or "humor." *Phlegmatic, sanguine, choleric,* and *melancholic* were the four personality types. If there was an imbalance in a humor, it caused disease and it was up to the healer to correct the deficiency or excess.

Since women, by nature, had a predominance of water in their bodies, their personalities were normally phlegmatic. When disease struck a woman, it usually robbed her of her phlegmatic properties, wetness and cold. If she was cursed with too much black bile, she became melancholic. The woman in Albrecht Dürer's *Melencolia I* evidently had a predominance of black bile.

---

tree, and I did eat."[3] Thus, the man was able to shirk responsibility for his act and blame the woman for his choices and actions. Then God told Eve, "I will greatly multiply thy sorrow and thy conception; in sorrow thou shalt bring forth children . . . and thy husband . . . he shall rule over thee"[4] (Figure 1).

Since that biblical time, women have suffered the consequences of these religious teachings and assumptions that have labeled their bodies as incomplete, inferior, and imperfect. As a corollary, women have been perceived as having less intelligence, a flawed mental structure, and no capacity for logical thought. One important result of this cultural assumption is that women's health care and participation in the medical system has been subordinate to, and different from, that of men's.

Biologically, the creation myth specified that it was the male rib which became the template for woman's entire body: "And Adam said, This *is* now bone of my bones and flesh of my flesh: she shall be called Woman, because she was taken out of Man."[5] Socially, however, it has been the muscular and soft tissue of the uterus, not the osseous tissue and cartilage, which have defined woman, her morality, personality, emotional makeup, and mental capacity. Yet other ideas about women, steeped in ancient humoral theory, remain under cover, disguised as science or unexamined in the wake of changing worldviews (Figure 2).

In cultures that did not or do not share our creation myth,

there is sorrow surrounding menstruation. In fact, many had rituals designed around rites of passage with regard to menarche (the first occurrence of menstruation), and each subsequent menstrual cycle. Certain Eskimo cultures tattooed girls on the chin to indicate they had experienced their first period, a mark of marriageability. According to Robert Spencer, "a menstruating woman was not allowed in the main chamber of the house . . . and women giving birth had to be secluded [because] they were offensive to the game, driving them away."[6] These cultural practices, though not as severe as in other Native American cultures, reflected the belief that "menstrual blood and postnatal flow were defiling and dangerous."[7] The Hupa of northwestern California required a girl to be isolated for ten days at the onset of visible signs of puberty because she was "considered unclean and her glance contaminating. . . . She was prohibited from eating meat or fresh fish and allowed to drink only warm water."[8] The Micmac in Nova Scotia built a lodge away from the main wigwam to house "women who had given birth and menstruating women," who were also "expected to eat from their own dishes."[9] They believed as well that "game would be offended if they came into contact, however it happened, with menstrual blood."[10]

All cultures create rules for their members with regard to work, play, speech, word usage, attire, social distance, body postures, gaze, and touch, as well as boundaries that limit where they can walk, run, eat, play sports, or worship. These rules are so woven into the fabric of a culture that most people do not question their logic. To a sophisticated audience, it may appear humorous that preliterate people held beliefs about pollution with regard to women's uterine functions. But before we criticize their ignorance, let's take a look at our own culture. A Miqwāh was recently unveiled in Boca Raton, Florida. This structure, built in an upwardly mobile, thoroughly modern community at a cost of more than two million dollars, is intended for the use of Jewish women who wish to ritually purify themselves after menstruation, and who pay big bucks for the privilege.[11]

Returning to the Old World will provide us with a fascinating history that links the pathology of both physical and mental diseases in women with the uterus. In ancient Egypt, a wandering womb was described in medical documents known as the Kahun and Smith papyri. Presumably the most ancient medical document, the Kahun (or Lahun, Illahun, or Kahoun) papyrus was almost exclusively dedicated to the issues of women's health care and the problems of the uterus, though it also addressed veterinary medicine. It was discovered near Cairo in 1889 by a British archeologist, Flinders Petrie, and reconstructed by Egyptologist F. L. Griffith. There were thirty-four sections to it. According to Dr. Clifford Snyder's *The Virtual Hospital,* the Kahun papyrus discussed such items as a falling womb, dysmenorrhea, and a wandering womb. (If not satisfied by sex or impregnation, the uterus was believed to leave its deep-seated place in the pelvis and search for that certain something somewhere else.) Some of the medicaments it advised were "incense, herbs, beer, goat's milk, and olive oil, vaginal fumigations, and other repulsive substances."[12] The Kahun papyrus dates approximately 2100–1900 B.C.E. and predates the Smith papyrus by two hundred years.

The Edwin Smith papyrus (circa 1700 B.C.E.) states that if a woman suffered in her abdomen, was unable to menstruate, or had trouble in the upper part of her vulva, she had an obstruction of the blood. The treatment prescribed was composed in part of one-sixteenth part wam, one-eighth part grease, and one-eighth part sweet beer, to be cooked and drunk for four days. (This leaves many unanswered questions. For example, of what was the remaining eleven-sixteenths of the formula composed? And how much was the patient supposed to drink?) The Smith papyrus also instructs the physician to mix an ointment of oil, tepnenet, eyepaint, and sweet frankincense, and to anoint the organ with this mixture very frequently.[13] Both the Kahun and Smith papyri are believed to have been copied from earlier works.

Etymologically, the Greek word for "womb" (*husteros*) meant "latter, lower," but its feminine form (*hustera*) "came to be applied specifically to the lower part of a woman's anatomy."[14] Since the wandering of the womb was believed to cause disease

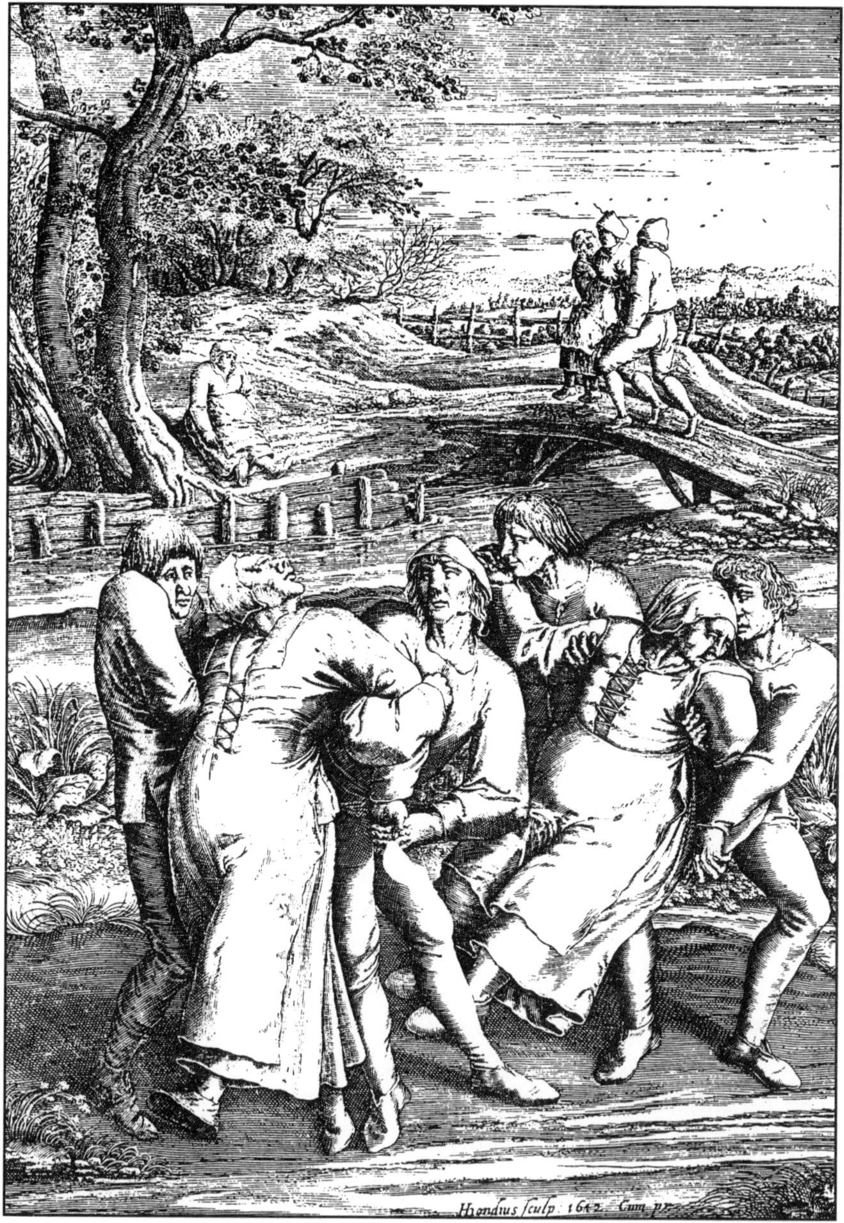

Two Groups of Epileptics Going to the Left, on page 130, in a book by H. Arthur Klein entitled *Graphic Worlds of Peter Bruegel the Elder,* 1963 Dover Publications, Inc. LC #63-17907.

Figure 3. **Hysteria Has Many Names and Faces.** Uterine hysteria was known by many names. One, *chorea lasciva,* was diagnosed by the German-Swiss alchemist and physician Philippus Paracelsus; it manifested itself in a dancing mania, a "dance which we find in whores and others who are not whores." Paracelsus wrote, "We have also to speak about the womb changed into an unfavorable one, which . . . results in a contraction of the uterus and takes away all reason. If the womb neither feels, nor has the proper substance, then it is cold. This causes . . . a sharp acid in the uterus. The contraction . . . and spasm also force the other limbs into spasms and tetanus, for they become contaminated by the womb also. If such contraction takes place in the veins of the whole body, vapor and smoke come out of the womb to the organs around it. And it touches the heart."

In this illustration by Peter Bruegel, women afflicted by uterine hysteria are restrained by men who will throw them into the water to cure their symptoms. (Cold water is a popular treatment for uncontrollable women, no matter in what century they present symptoms.) Their enlarged abdomens are the result of "sour uterine vapors," a cause of hysteria. The vapors remained a cause of illness in women for approximately four hundred more years.

Paracelsus lived from 1493 to 1541. He did not subscribe to the humoral theory and based his treatments on specific remedies. Peter Bruegel (1530–1569) attempted to illustrate *chorea lasciva* or hysteria, but it wasn't until 1642 that his drawings were found, then engraved by Henrick Hondius.

---

in women, "hysteria" became a catch-all term for a variety of female illnesses and behaviors. Even a great scholar like Hippocrates was unable to keep from getting confused. He used his excellent clinical description of epilepsy synonymously with hysteria, though he "maintained the uterine origin [of hysteria] and strictly excluded it from the category of mental disease"[15] (Figure 3). Since then, many more great minds have shared in the confusion with regard to women, hysteria, and normality. Even Sigmund Freud, the founder of modern psychology, "elaborated melancholia or pathological mourning, as a form of hysteria."[16]

A peculiar contradiction developed because, although the sexually unsatisfied uterus was diagnosed as the reason for women's health problems, the recognition or expression of sexuality was viewed as an abnormal attribute in women. In fact, at various times in history, to be sexual was to put oneself in the precarious position of being diagnosed as a witch or as having

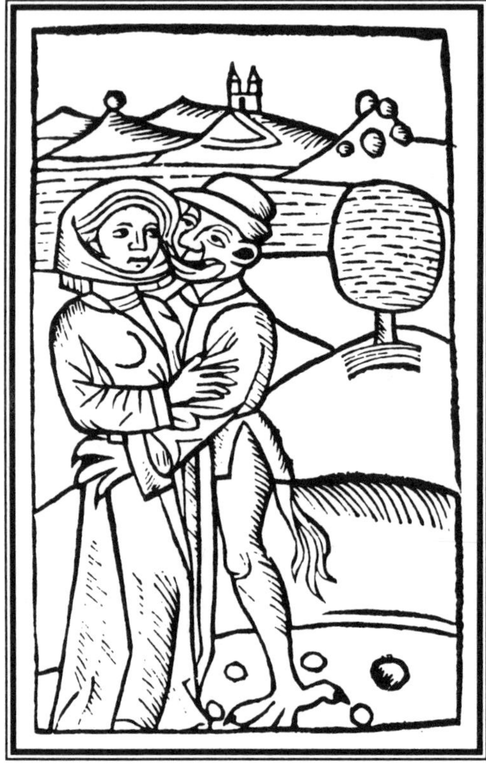

From Ulrifig Molitor's *Von den Unholden und Hexen,* Constance, 1489. Courtesy of Dover Pictorial Archive Series.

***Figure 4.* Requirements for a Witch.** A witch must have a female body. She must have a skin tag hidden in a secret place where the devil can suck on her. She must be sexually insatiable and weak in character. If these qualities are present, she is qualified to be a witch and liable to be seduced by the devil. As Sibylle Harksen observes in *Women in the Middle Ages,* the belief in witches and witchcraft would ultimately account "for as many victims as the persecution of heretics . . . although the Church at first did not give credence to" these notions.

---

consort with the devil (Figure 4). The bodies of suspect women were scrupulously searched for special anatomical parts called "witches' tits." These appendages, not always obvious to initial scrutiny, were "proof" that sexual congress with the devil could be achieved (Figure 5). They were described by the various "experts" of the days as "divers strange marks, at which (as som of them have confessed) the Devill sucks their bloud,"[17] and as "a preternatural excrescence of flesh between the pudendum and anus, much like to teats, and not usual in women."[18] Searching for these evil marks, as well as torturing confessions out of women and then punishing them for their witchcraft, were all energetic functions of the church, which used medical examinations to confirm its diagnosis.

As society vigorously pursued women in search of their hidden fleshy skin tags, by the sixteenth and seventeenth centuries a tremendous paradigm shift had taken place. Care of the uterus had previously and traditionally been exclusively in the sphere of women, midwives who attended births. No formal gynecology existed, even though a few late Renaissance documents were produced, such as *Thrésor des remèdes secrets pour les maladies des femmes* (*Treasury of Secret Remedies for Women's Diseases*). Another expert of the day, Arnaud de Villeneuve, explained his *Practica* when he wrote, "With the help of God I shall here concern myself with matters having to do with women, and since women are most of the time vicious animals, I shall in due course consider the bite of venomous animals."[19] Because female health problems were perceived as frightening, and pregnancy as pathologic, the doctors who had begun to practice obstetrics wanted to control the suffering and the changes they perceived as the disturbed physiology of pregnancy. There was a certain irony to this: As Evelyne Berriot-Salvadore has observed, "In this respect medical discourse appears to have been at odds with Christian morality which condemned women to give birth in pain."[20] But as men gained permission to treat women's obstetrical conditions, women's skills to do the same were correspondingly devalued. Midwifery, a family tradition handed down from mother to daughter through many generations, became the subject of troublesome restrictions. One example is provided by historian Merry Wiesner in the judgment handed down against a German medical practitioner in 1598 by the Memmingen City Council: "Elizabeth Heyssin is to be allowed to treat external wounds and sores in the same manner that she has been doing up till now, but only on women and children when they request it of her . . . her daughter, though, is to be totally forbidden from practicing any kind of medicine."[21] As European societies pushed to marginalize folk knowledge, professional training grew. By 1560, a formal program in midwifery was established in Paris which required the approval of licensed physicians and midwives for licensure.

From Henry Gray, *Anatomy of the Human Body,* 22nd ed. (Philadelphia and New York: Lea & Febiger, 1930).

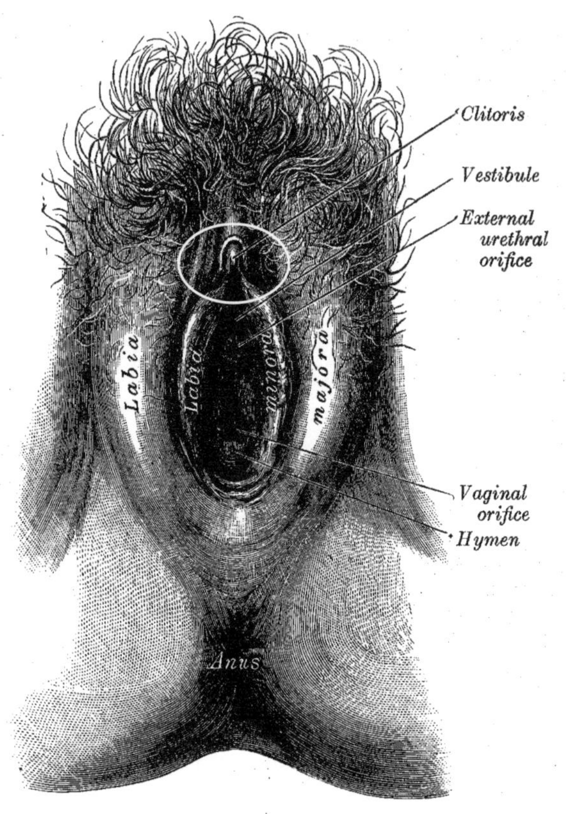

Still, if a man were present in the lying-in room, he was usually the husband of the woman in labor.

Interestingly, at one point the Bible was used to oppose male entry into the midwifery profession. Jane Sharp, an English midwife who wrote *The Compleat Midwife's Companion,* contested man's place in the delivery room because female midwives were sanctioned by the Bible whereas male midwives were not. Both the College of Surgeons and the College of Physicians had different reasons for not wanting men to be midwives, but there were also physicians who argued against women upgrading their status with formal education. According to Lois Magner, "Dr. Samuel Merriman, Physician to Middlesex Hospital, argued that women were totally unable to master scientific knowledge or use medical instruments."[22]

***Figure 5.* A Witch's Tit.** Two of the foremost witch-hunters of the fifteenth century were Jacob Sprenger and Heinrich Kramer, who described their discovery of the witch's tit as follows: "We find, on her secret parts, growing within the lip of the same, a loose piece of skin and when pulled it is near an inch long [and] somewhat in form of the finger of a glove flattened." (Quoted by Paul Boyar and Stephen Nissenbaum in their book *Salem Possessed: The Social Origins of Witchcraft.*)

The English equivalents of Sprenger and Kramer were the Witch Finder General, Matthew Hopkins, and his assistant, John Sterne. According to Richard Deacon in his book *Matthew Hopkins: Witch Finder General,* the pair executed eighteen witches at Bury St. Edmunds because they " 'were found by the searchers to have teats or dugs which their imps used to suck.' Most of these supernumerary teats were located in the labia majora. More often than not what was alleged to have been a 'Devil's mark' was no more than a well-developed and swollen clitoris."

At a witch trial in 1593, according to Barbara G. Walker in *The Women's Encyclopedia of Myths and Secrets,* the investigating jailer, a married man, apparently discovered a clitoris for the first time. Barbara Rosen, in her book *Witchcraft,* quotes a contemporary account: "After the execution was ended . . . and three persons were thoroughly dead, the jailer stripped off their clothes and, being naked, he found upon the body of the old woman Alice Samuel a little lump of flesh, in manner sticking out as if it had been a teat to the length of half an inch; which both he and his wife perceiving, at the first sight thereof meant not to disclose because it was adjoining to so secret a place which was not decent to be seen. Yet in the end, not willing to conceal so strange a matter, and decently covering that privy place a little above which it grew, they made open show thereof."

Opponents of male midwifery countered by raising the issue of corrupted female virtue. The preservation of modesty was an important consideration; how could any self-respecting husband allow another male to know his wife in such an intimate way? According to Philip Thicknesse, "One argument was that a woman handled by the man-midwife became polluted [and] more likely to admit other men to similar familiarities."[23] Despite all the controversy, males gained access, though guarded, to control of the fecund uterus. Because moral obstacles had historically prohibited males from the birthing room, sometimes a male doctor had to crawl into the room on all fours, unseen by the laboring women. (In a few cases, men even disguised themselves as women.) The most significant change, however, is attributed to the use of obstetrical forceps, developed over a period between 1600 and 1728 by Peter Chamberlen the Elder and his heirs, all practicing male midwives. The technology of forceps use would have a powerful effect on how the uterus was controlled after the eighteenth century.

Throughout the eighteenth century, hysteria still hovered in the body parts of virgins, wives, and widows. More than a vestige of humoral theory was apparent in the work of R. James, M.D., who informed physicians that if their female patients were "full of blood and moisture and have not borne children," the cure, like in ancient times, was "to be expected from marriage. Reason, Experience and the Authorities of the greatest Physicians, concur in pronouncing Matrimony highly beneficial in removing hysteric Disorders."[24]

By the nineteenth century, the transition from midwives to doctors was almost complete, although "the proper Victorian lady was expected to prefer death to a discussion of gynecological problems with a male physician."[25] Unfortunately, the clinical experience that enabled doctors to learn more about the uterus dealt a tragic blow to those who dared to trust them. Puerperal fever, an iatrogenic disease, would infect and kill hundreds of women in the eighteenth and nineteenth centuries. Even after the avenues of infection had been identified, women still suffered because men didn't want to wash their hands.

By the nineteenth century, hysteria had moved from the uterus to the brain; and although no one still believed that the uterus could travel toward the head, the shift from somatic to psychologic etiology did not free women from the control of the male medical establishment. Now, an "unstable" woman could be incarcerated in an institution or labeled "melancholic," "insane," or "nymphomaniac" if she did not fulfill her husband's or society's expectations. Moreover, female behavior could be attributed to uterine proclivities. Doctors were able to aid troubled husbands who were uninformed about female sexuality. Surgical procedures such as clitoridectomy and ovariotomy were touted as cures for unnatural female behavior. These operations did silence or subdue many an unruly female, sometimes with a thank you from the patient.

As if punishment for menstruation, sexual desire, and pregnancy were not enough, the pejorative and even hostile attitudes toward women as a result of their uterine ownership has limited female participation in the mainstream of life's nonbiological creativity. Education, particularly university education, was difficult to obtain for most women until the twentieth century. The nineteenth-century stories of three women attempting to obtain their doctorates in medicine—Marie Zakrzewska, Harriot Hunt, and Elizabeth Blackwell—demonstrate a persistent struggle to succeed and magnify the women's health issues of the time in their fight to be legitimized as physicians.

During the twentieth century, a full-fledged war over control of the uterus has erupted in such issues as compulsory caesarean sections, sterilization of the "unfit," medicalization of childbirth, wholesale hysterectomy, illegal abortion, and surrogate motherhood. Ironically, the uterus—whose possession historically has caused women to be labeled as inferior, invalid, and insane—became the fertile ground for contemporary political tugs of war.

Although science has progressed in understanding uterine anatomy (as well as the egalitarian statistical distribution of intelligence and the limitations of sex hormones on personality), all too many women are still kept subject to unexamined cultural survivals. My goal in this book is to exhume the origins of those ideas, carefully arrange them on the dissection table, inject them with humor, and prosect them under a new light.

Endnotes

1. Peggy Sanday, *Female Power and Male Dominance: The Origins of Sexual Inequality* (New York: Cambridge University Press, 1981), p. 16.
2. Genesis 3:6.
3. Genesis 3:11.

4. Genesis 3:16.

5. Genesis 2:23.

6. Robert Spencer et al., *The Native Americans: Ethnology and Backgrounds of the North American Indians* (New York: Harper and Row, 1977), p. 89.

7. Ibid., p. 211.

8. Ibid., p. 371.

9. Ibid.

10. Ibid.

11. "Synagogue Building Bath," Fort Lauderdale *Sun Sentinel* (December 23, 1993); "Temple Briefs—Dedication," Fort Lauderdale *Sun Sentinel* (November 25, 1994).

12. Clifford Snyder, *The Virtual Hospital* (Internet document: 1995). http://vh.radiology.viowa.edu/Provi.textbooks/SnyderMedHx/020Papyrihtml.

13. Otto Bettmann, *A Pictorial History of Medicine* (Springfield, Ill.: Charles C. Thomas, 1972), p. 6.

14. Jane Mills, *Womanwords: A Dictionary of Words About Women* (New York: Henry Holt and Company), 1989, p. 123.

15. Ilza Veith, *Hysteria: The History of a Disease* (Chicago: University of Chicago Press, 1965), p. 14.

16. Mary Burgan, *Illness, Gender, and Writing* (Baltimore: Johns Hopkins University Press, 1994), p. 90.

17. Quoted in Michael Macdonald, *Witchcraft and Hysteria in Elizabethan London: Edward Jorden and the Mary Glover Case* (New York: Tavistock/Routledge, 1991), p. 28.

18. Quoted in Paul Boyar and Stephen Nissenbaum, *Salem Possessed: The Social Origins of Witchcraft* (Cambridge: Harvard University Press, 1974), p. 13.

19. Quoted in Evelyne Berriot-Salvadore, "The Discourse of Medicine and Science." In Georges Duby and Michelle Perrot, eds., *A History of Women in the West, Volume 3: Renaissance and Enlightenment Paradoxes* (Cambridge: Belknap Press, 1993), p. 350.

20. Berriot-Salvadore, p. 379.

21. Quoted in Margaret L. King, *Women of the Renaissance* (Chicago: University of Chicago Press, 1991), p. 46.

22. Lois Magner, *A History of Medicine* (New York: Marcel Dekker, Inc., 1992), p. 273.

23. Quoted in Jean Donnison, *Midwives and Medical Men* (London: Heinemann, 1977), p. 30.

24. Quoted in Vivien Jones, ed., *Women in the Eighteenth Century* (London: Routledge, 1990), p. 86.

25. Magner, p. 274.

CHAPTER 1
Ancient Themes

Hysteria. The origin of this quintessential "female problem" may date back as far as circa 2000 B.C.E., after an observant Egyptian midwife palpated a prolapsed uterus and declared, "It's a fallen womb." Logically, if the uterus could unhinge and fall out of the pelvis, it could go up as well—or anywhere. As it did, the movement of this organ could cause a variety of illnesses in women, according to an ancient work known as the Kahun papyrus. This wandering womb, in its search for satisfaction, slammed into the liver, punched the stomach, and crushed the spleen, causing pain. The uterus also compressed the lungs, stifled the breath, and caused suffocation. While the afflicted woman gasped for air, her associates scrambled in all directions to search for some herbs to burn, fanning the fumes toward her head or feet. Asphyxia was one symptom of hysteria, and its treatment was limited to aromatherapy.

The Ebers papyrus, a medical document similar to the Kahun and Smith papyri, had specialized information only for

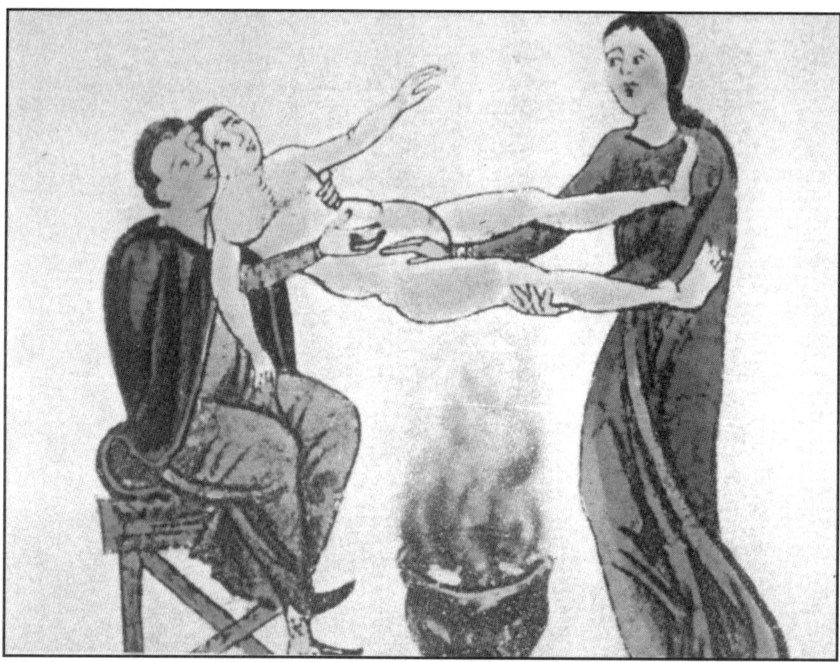

***Figure 6.* One Treatment for a Wandering Womb.** When the womb wandered toward the head, noxious-smelling substances were burned near the nose to repel the uterus. Then fragrant and pleasing fumes of aromatic substances were directed toward the vulva. This would assist to lure the uterus down into the pelvis, where it belonged. This figure shows a medieval image of the Egyptian practice. Private collection.

the treatment of women's ailments. As Ilza Veith reports, one therapy for a uterus that would not hold still was for the patient to "sit on a roll of cloth that had been moistened with the dregs of an infusion of pine sawdust." Noxious drinks were also prescribed: "A . . . potion composed of tar from the wood of a ship and the dregs of beer, was supposed, by its evil taste, to induce the descent of the uterus."[1] Wandering wombs were treated from both ends. Ancient Egyptian healers burned substances above and below the pelvis. The smoke near the head was intentionally malodorous; this would repel the uterus, sending it downward. Then a bowl of aromatic substances would be placed on the ground under the woman's spread legs. These

Courtesy of the Brooklyn Museum of Art.

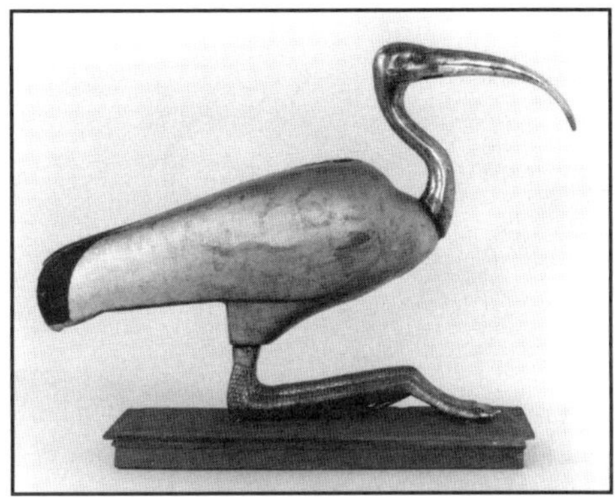

Figure 7. **Thoth.** The Egyptians believed that medical lore originated with the gods, particularly Thoth, the god of healing who took the earthly form of an ibis. In many belief systems, a supernatural deity takes the natural form of an animal. A wax model of this bird was used by the Egyptians to insert in the vagina and force the womb back to its place. Its functional beak could impart medications to many orifices. The apocryphal invention of the enema is attributed to the long-beaked ibis, which penetrated its cloaca in order to administer medicine.

---

pleasing and fragrant vapors were supposed to lure the uterus downward (Figure 6). An alternate therapy was dried excrement of men placed on frankincense. Certain writers insisted that the definitive treatment had to include a male component; if the uterus was unhappy because it had not received enough male substance, only something masculine would cure it. If conception was desired, a plaintive call to the supernatural was made to Thoth, who allegedly had magical powers of healing (Figure 7).

The Greek philosopher Plato called the uterus an animal within an animal and argued that it was a major cause of young women's health problems. If it was deprived of sexual activity or was barren for too long, the disgruntled uterus would exit the pelvic basin in search of satisfaction. In doing so, it would wreak havoc on other organ systems. As Plato stated in *Timaeus*:

> In females, what is called the womb or uterus is like a living thing, possessed of the desire to make children. . . . The womb

> is an animal which longs to generate children. When it remains barren too long after puberty, it is distressed and sorely disturbed, and straying about in the body and cutting off the passages of the breath, it impedes respiration and brings the sufferer into the extremest anguish and provokes all manner of diseases besides.[2]

"Such," he concluded, "is the nature of women and all that is female."

But Hippocrates, the ancient Greek physician, strongly disagreed (Figure 8). He called it *globus hystericus* and diagnosed it primarily in older women:

> Prolonged continence was believed to result in demonstrable organic changes in the womb. . . . [I]n such situations, the uterus dries up and loses weight and in its search for moisture, rises toward the hypochondrium, thus impeding the flow of breath which was supposed normally to descend into the abdominal cavity. If the organ comes to rest in this position, it causes convulsions similar to those of epilepsy."[3]

Not so, wrote Aretaeus, the second-century physician who is ranked just below Hippocrates in the importance of his contributions to medicine. Aretaeus concurred with Plato that young women had peregrinations of the uterus: "In the middle of the flanks of women, lies the womb, a female viscus in the flanks . . . closely resembling an animal; for it is moved of itself hither and thither and, in a word, it is altogether erratic."[4] He advised young women to find a sex partner as quickly as possible to keep their uteruses under control.

Meanwhile, Galen, the Greek anatomist, physician, and author, had his own views on the subject, writing that "the man is more perfect than the woman, [who is] less perfect than the man in respect to the generative parts." In Galen's schema, a uterus was an inverted scrotum: "The parts were formed within her when she was still a fetus, but could not, because of the defect in the heat, emerge and project on the outside." Galen

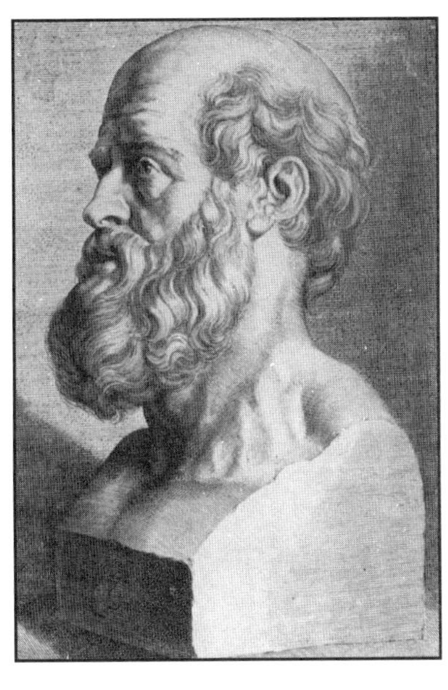

Figure 8. **Hippocrates.** Many images have been rendered to represent Hippocrates, yet this popular one is probably not as accurate as a less handsome representation. During the time of Hippocrates, it was believed that the fetus swam out of the uterus when ready. Hippocrates taught that the womb wandered around in a woman's body, causing disease as a consequence of its impact on other tissues.

Among his other teachings were that a premature baby was more viable at seven than at eight months of age, and that females were produced from semen from the left ovary. Hippocrates did, however, write some accurate descriptions of authentic gynecological problems.

The Hippocratic Oath attributed to the so-called Father of Medicine mandates that a physician should not give a woman an abortifacient nor engage in sexual relations with female patients. But according to Albert Lyons and R. Joseph Petrucelli in their book *Medicine: An Illustrated History,* although the Hippocratic Oath has been taken by multitudes of medical students throughout the ages, its rules may not actually have been part of Hippocratic philosophy.

---

went on to explain that because of this lack of heat, the would-be scrotum remained inside, which meant that women had semen just like men, but if they went without sex for too long, the "seed" would accumulate and cause hysteria (Figure 9). Women who had long been accustomed to sexual activity were particularly susceptible to this repression of germinal matter or spoiled seed. Ostensibly, marriage guaranteed sexual activity for uteruses, young and old alike. Or as Galen himself put it, "You ought not to think that our Creator would purposely make half the whole race imperfect and, as it were, mutilated, unless there was some great advantage in such a mutilation."

Galen deserves credit for knowing enough about anatomy to realize that the diaphragm, a sturdy sheet of muscle which separates the thoracic cavity from the abdominal viscera, would

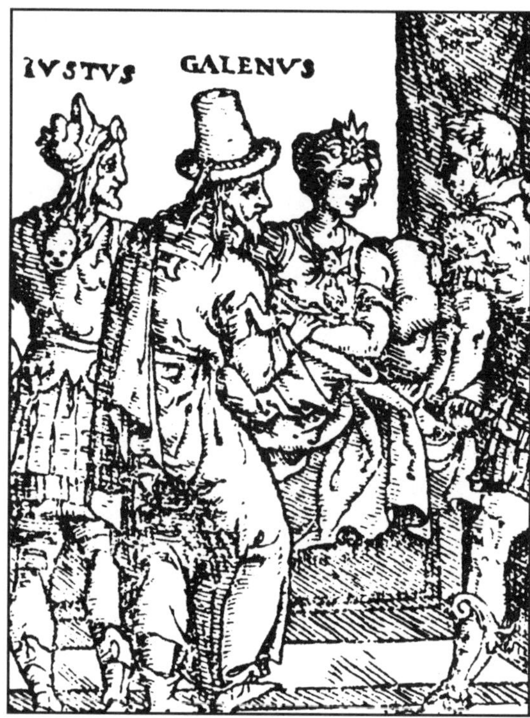

***Figure 9.* Galen's Diagnostic Acumen.** Galen (130–201 C.E.) was the Greek physician who wrote that man was more perfect than woman because his genitalia were external. According to the humoral theory, a woman's genitalia were inside her body because she lacked the heat necessary for their emergence. Galen endorsed this model, but he was perspicacious enough to recognize that sometimes a young woman's ailments were due to lovesickness rather than physical causes. He was also wise enough to recognize that men, too, suffered from it.

---

not allow the uterus to travel past its superior border. Despite this insight, Galen nevertheless perpetuated the diagnostic category of *hysterical suffocation.* This is not surprising; as Thomas Kuhn has famously observed, "Normal science often suppresses fundamental novelties because they are necessarily subversive of its basic commitments."[5] It would be many years after Galen's era that science would dare to publish revolutionary new information about the human body, overturning many of the ancient concepts that Galen used to treat his patients. In his eyes, hysterical suffocation affected "those who have previously menstruated regularly, had been pregnant and were eager to have intercourse, but were now deprived of all this." This deprivation resulted in repressed menstrual flow which in turn "caused the uterine condition by which . . . women become . . . suffocated or spastic."[6] *Suffocation of the mother* became a new term, one that would be echoed throughout the centuries. And although everyone knew the cure for suffocation was to restore normal sexual function to these deprived women, the ways for women without partners to achieve this were not spelled out in any detail. Indeed, although unmarried sex was not clearly defined as evil in Galen's time, the day when it would be forbidden was soon to come.

Endnotes

1. Ilza Veith, *Hysteria: The History of a Disease* (Chicago: University of Chicago Press, 1965), p. 5.
2. Claude Thomasset, "The Nature of Woman." In *A History of Women in the West, Volume 2: Silences of the Middle Ages,* Georges Duby and Michelle Perrot, eds. (Cambridge: Belknap Press, 1992), p. 48; Veith, pp. 7–8.
3. Veith, p. 10.
4. Quoted in Phillip R. Slavney, *Perspectives on Hysteria* (Baltimore: Johns Hopkins University Press, 1990), pp. 13–14.
5. Thomas Kuhn, *The Structure of Scientific Revolutions* (Chicago: University of Chicago Press, 1967), p. 5.
6. Slavney, p. 15.

Chapter 2
Eve's Legacy

Do you know that each of you women is an Eve? The sentence of God on this sex of yours lives in this age; the guilt must necessarily live too. You are the gate of Hell, you are the temptress of the forbidden tree; you are the first deserter of the divine law.

—Tertullian[1]

Unfortunately, early Judeo-Christian thinkers created a set of rules that precluded help for the problems which plagued women as a result of their errant uteri. Western religion could no longer endorse the known cures for women's ailments because they challenged the principles of virginity, chastity, and abstinence. To satisfy a hungry uterus and restore health via sexual satisfaction was just not acceptable. The days of appeasement by passion and love were over. In fact, any erotic thoughts, feelings, knowledge, or expression were strictly forbidden. As Arno Karlen points out, "Christianity expressed obsessively and frantically the idea that woman and sex are pollutions, barriers to religious grace."[2] Women were to remain virgins until marriage—or, in the absence of marriage, forever. This was the opinion held by many major writers of the time, who produced a number of books in praise of virginity. Among the treatises dealing with women written in the first seven centuries are *On the Wearing of Veils by Virgins* by Tertullian, *On the Conduct of Virgins* by Cyprian, *On the True Integrity of Virginity* by Basil of Ancyra, *On Virgins* by Ambrose of Milan, *On Holy Virginity* by Augustine, *Forty-Sixth Letter to a Fallen Virgin* by Basil of Caesaria, and *On the Fall of a Consecrated Virgin* by Niceta of Remesiana.

If this seems excessive, we have Augustine to thank for the fallout from the ridiculous opinions he expressed in his *Confessions.* His writings not only denied sexual activity (the cure for a wandering womb) to widows, nuns, and unmarried women, but conjugal pleasure to married women as well. (Which is to say that Augustine permitted married people to have sex, but they weren't supposed to enjoy it.) Indeed, Augustine felt that "carnal pleasures were the work of unholy spirits" and wrote in his *Soliloquies,* "Nothing is so much to be shunned as sex relations."[3] At least he didn't discriminate, urging men to forego sex as well as women.

Augustine's plea for celibacy can best be explained by inspecting and analyzing his own personal philosophical journey. At age seventeen, he entered into a sexual relationship with a woman whom he impregnated. According to Uta Ranke-Heinemann, he observed his "partner's infertile days although his vigilance was frustrated by a miscalculation that blessed him with Adeodatus [his son]."[4] Augustine's Christian mother, St. Monica, sternly criticized her son's choice of lover, lifestyle, and even religion. In his youth, Augustine embraced Manichaenism, a syncretic sect which believed

> the god of Light had sent Jesus in the form of the Incarnate Word to warn Adam that Eve was the tool of darkness, and as a result Adam refused to sleep with her. The powers of darkness countered this refusal by teaching Eve the necessary

> witchcraft by which she seduced Adam so that he became her mate and together they propagated the world.[5]

The Manichees believed that procreation was evil, marriage was a sin, and proteinaceous food (food that resulted from sexual reproduction) was taboo. Augustine was able to survive in this milieu because the Manichees recognized that not all people could adhere to such ascetic standards and forego pleasure, sex, and meat. Manichaenism therefore had a triple-ranked hierarchy: "The true Manichaen adherents were the Adepts, those who had been able to tame concupiscence and covetousness, to refrain from eating flesh, and to refuse to have sexual intercourse. Those who believed in the teaching of Mani [their savior] but were not yet Adepts were Auditors, men and women of goodwill but who could not yet contain themselves, but were trying to do so."[6] The lowest rung was occupied by everyone else, the populace-at-large that was hopelessly lacking a belief in Mani and so embraced sensuality and evil.

Augustine was an Auditor. His mother was not too happy with this; she was something of a social climber and had chosen a bride from a "good family" for him. In fact, she pressured her son so effectively to break off his relationship that Augustine finally banished his mistress from their home. Unfortunately, the bride his mother had chosen was still under age, and during the two years that Augustine was forced to wait for her to mature, he underwent severe psychological stress: "To a large extent what held me captive and tortured me was the habit of satisfying with vehement intensity an insatiable sexual desire," he states in the *Confessions.* He took up with yet another woman, and his justification for doing so was that he felt helpless against his carnal desires. In what Freudian psychoanalysis would call a reaction formation, he suddenly converted to Christianity and chose celibacy over pleasure, neither marrying the girl his mother had chosen nor remaining with his interim girlfriend.

According to Vern and Bonnie Bullough, "Though he then rose rapidly in the Christian hierarchy, Augustine carried with him many of his Manichaen ideas about sex. Perhaps inevitably, sexual intercourse for Augustine came to be regarded as the greatest threat to spiritual freedom."[7] Christianity stressed virginity, but sexual relations were allowed so long as they conformed to certain restrictions: They had to be performed within a marital bond, in the correct position (male above, female below, the classic "missionary position"), for the purpose of procreation, and motivated by God's will rather than a desire for human pleasure. Any variation from these standards was considered sinful and deviant.

As a result of this early male domination, Vern Bullough writes, "misogynism became ingrained in Christianity."[8] Perhaps if more women had participated in the formulation of the "rules" of the church, celebration rather than disdain would have characterized the founders' attitudes. As it was, women did not participate enough in the literature to have any influence. They were not only forbidden to teach in the church but were required to be silent.[9] The rationale for this was simple: In the New Testament, there were no female apostles.

During Augustine's lifetime, an important medical work, Soranus's *On Diseases of Women,* was preserved (albeit in fragments) in the writings of Oribasius. By the sixth century, Muscio had abstracted part of the manuscript in Latin and, by 850 C.E., a drawing based on Muscio's translation was included in another manuscript (Figure 10). Perhaps if the entire opus had been available, the myth of the wandering uterus would have been put to rest forever, but it wasn't until the Renaissance that more of Soranus's knowledge became available, and it wasn't until the nineteenth century that Western culture retrieved the complete wisdom of his writings.

Meanwhile, midwives took care of the uterus. In all cultures and throughout history, women have been healers. Western European cultures depended on female healers, known as "wise women" or "midwives," who possessed folk knowledge disseminated through oral tradition of medicinal plants and herbs, as well as ways to prepare and administer them. Women

Muscio's 850 C.E. interpretation of the uterus from the writings of Soranus. From a manuscript of about 850 C.E. in the Royal Library at Brussels (MS. 3714, folio 16). Reprinted by permission of Dover Publications, Inc.

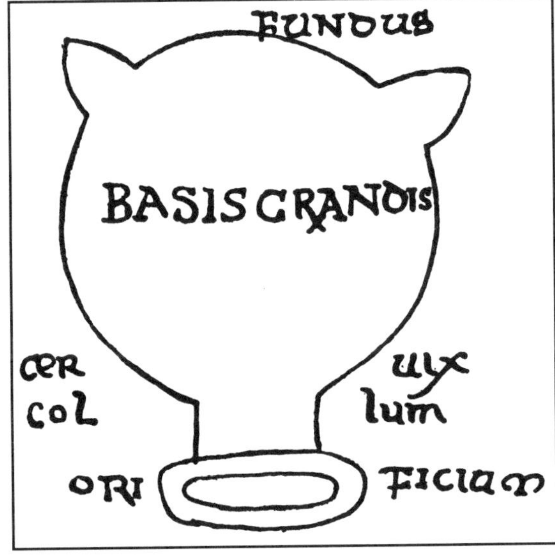

Figure 10. **The Cat-Headed Uterus of Soranus.** One of the earliest documents about the uterus was written by Soranus. His writings have been translated many times into various languages. As a result of these varying translations, different eras have represented the uterus in a variety of ways, all of them based on Soranus's work.

aided women during pregnancy, childbirth, menopause, and with other health issues. At times they provided health care to men as well. It is believed that some administered analgesics during labor and could perform abortions and advise on contraception. But as Christianity grew, the roles these women performed were increasingly regulated. According to Edward Shorter, by the thirteenth century "the Church's main concern was that the midwives administer emergency baptism according to the correct formulas, if they thought the infant was not going to survive the passage into the outside world."[10]

While the church kept its eye on midwives in individual communities, it also sought control over distant people whose views differed from its own. According to Sibylle Harksen, "From the twelfth century onwards heretical movements began increasingly to worry the Church,"[11] while Jeffrey Burton Russell notes that "in many of these movements, women were more respected than was usual for the period."[12] One of these heretical groups, the Cathari, was particularly attractive to women because of its egalitarian views. Women could act as priests as well as earn money within this sect. Interestingly, the Cathari had much in common with the Manichees: They had levels of membership, the Perfecti and the Credentes, as well as a belief that the soul, which came from the "kingdom of light," sought relief through the body, perceived as the "kingdom of darkness." Certain communities, exclusively comprised of women, performed necessary tasks like spinning and nursing the sick. Some members even educated the daughters of the nobility. In order to counteract this growing display of independence, the church established a convent in Prouille, France, which took in converts from Catharism. When this effort was less than successful, the church turned to more radical methods. "The last stronghold of the Cathari was the castle-fortress of Montségur. After its conquest in 1244, 200 men and women were burned at the stake."[13]

Religious movements that allowed women more rights, such as the Cathari, the *Pauperes Christi,* and the followers of John Huss, posed a serious challenge to (and were perceived as synonymous with heresy by) the patriarchal authority of the church. The results were predictably bloody. As Sibylle Harksen has argued, "The belief in witchcraft accounted for as many victims as the persecution of heretics. Belief in the devil gave rise in the early Middle Ages to the concept of witches" (although interestingly, as Harksen notes, "the Church at first did not give credence to this notion").[14] And according to Jeffrey Burton Russell, "While popes and Inquisitors were solidifying the legal and theoretical amalgamation of witchcraft with heresy, the witch phenomenon continued in practice to draw upon actual heresy."[15] The model of the witch evolved from a set of innocuous ideas about village healers and their control over nature and eventually culminated in the holocaust of many women in the sixteenth and seventeenth centuries (Figure 11).

According again to Russell, there was an amalgamation of several traditions which formed the concept of the witch: night vampires who drank human blood, Valkyries who played their games in the air, a fear of ghosts walking about at night, and the "wild ride."[16] Witches were accused of "night flying, secret meetings, harmful magic, and the devil's pact," which Sigrid Brauner points out were all "ascribed individually or in limited combinations by the church to its adversaries, including Templars, heretics, learned magicians, and other dissident groups."[17] An additional characteristic of witches was their predilection for flesh, especially children's flesh. Bishops were instructed to "drive out of their dioceses those who believe in and practice the wild ride. . . . The sentence of exile was justified on the grounds that those who practice these things have implicitly cut themselves off from God and become heretics and servants of the Devil."[18] And so the stage was set for the punishment of women believed to be heretics or witches. As Vern Bullough points out,

> Until almost the thirteenth century the official position of the Christian church was that acts associated with witchcraft were all illusions or fantasies originating in dreams and that belief in the actuality of witches was a pagan and heretical custom. This idea was challenged in the writings of St. Thomas Aquinas, who held that even though witches might be illusions or dreams they were no less real.[19]

Early attributions of witchcraft had much to do with the fertility of crops and animals as well as people. Control was closely related to nature and resources; the witch "destroys cattle, spreads mysterious diseases, makes men impotent, kills and eats infants, steals milk and butter and raises disastrous storms."[20] A witch could also sell unbaptized souls to the devil, thus making a dead newborn more valuable than a live birth (Figure 12). The uterus could miscarry or fail to become impregnated if a witch willed it. Later, the sexual, seductive, and

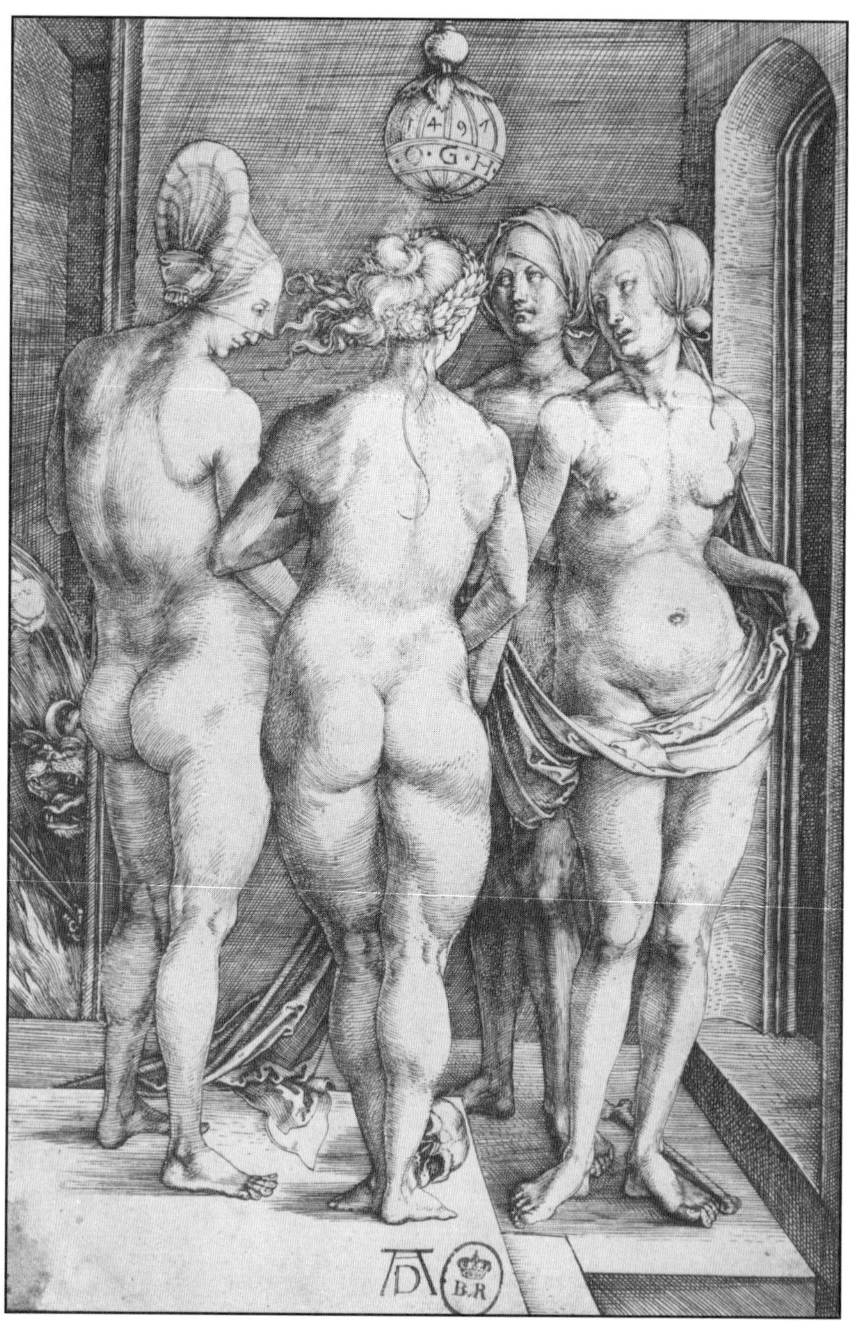

Albrecht Dürer (1471–1528). *The Four Witches.* 1497. Engraving (B. 75). Courtesy of the Bibliothèque Nationale, Paris, France. Giraudon/Art Resource, NY.

***Figure 11.* Witches Discuss Their Many Evils.** Witches come in many shapes and sizes, from the haggard, hunch-backed, broom-flying, edentulous, warty crone to the sensual, *zaftig,* fertile, and fecund seductress. According to Barbara Ehrenreich and Deidre English, the healer/wise woman was a role closely associated with the concept of the witch. Because illness was a punishment for evil, only God could choose to heal. Therefore, if a woman demonstrated that she could heal, it was believed her power came from the devil. In the traditions of the early church, God would not give women such power.

---

promiscuous qualities of witches became more salient features; then Renaissance thought would promote the idea that witches were women more often than men because women were so lascivious that they would more easily fall prey to temptation.

Throughout it all, the nature of females—defined by the weakness of body and mind—served as the underlying theme. According to Vern Bullough and James Brundage, medieval canon lawyers

> strongly believed that the sexuality of women differed from that of men, since women had not been created in the image of God as a man was, but out of a rib of man to serve as his companion and helpmate. This lesser creation, so to speak, made women more susceptible to sexual temptations, and their chastity, therefore, was more likely to be suspect. . . . [Husbands therefore] had a moral obligation to keep their wives sexually satisfied lest they be tempted to stray to other beds.[21]

It was apparently a losing battle. The age abounded in images of female evil likely to create anxiety, particularly in men isolated from day-to-day experience with (or knowledge of) women. When members of a society are removed from regular contact with the opposite sex, they will form fantasies based on speculation and fear about the unknowable and the unfathomable. As Brother William declares in *The Name of the Rose,* Umberto Eco's fictionalized recreation of life in a medieval monastery:

> And of woman as source of temptation the Scriptures have already said enough. Ecclesiastes says of woman that her con-

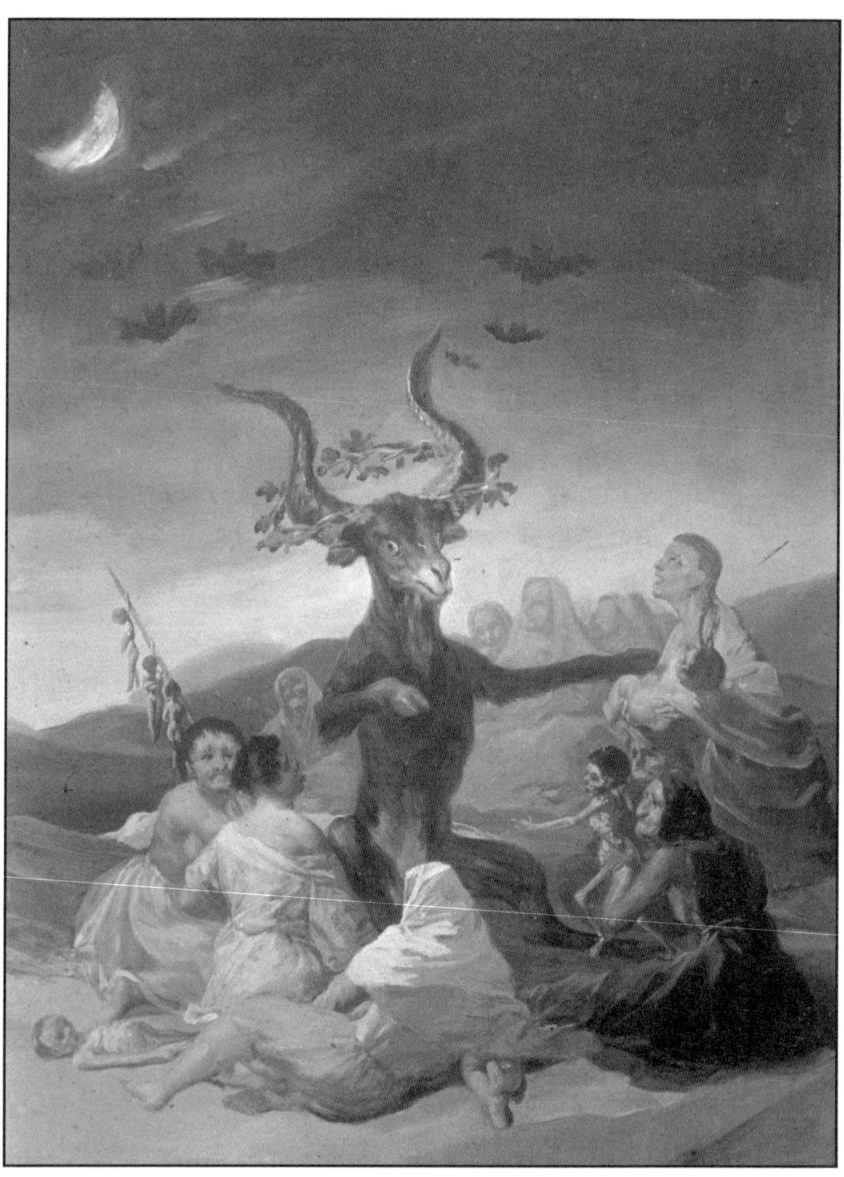

Francisco de Goya y Lucientes. *Witches Sabbath.* Museo Lazaro Galdiano, Madrid, Spain. Scala/Art Resource, NY.

Figure 12. **Midwives Sell the Souls of Dead Babies.** A *liminal* event is one fraught with uncertainty and indecision because it occurs between two life-stages or changes. In addition, liminal experiences are the subject of much superstition. Childbirth and death are liminal experiences; they are transitional in that a new life comes into the world and an established life leaves it. Wherever such passages take place, great anxiety is expended in dealing with them. Most societies create rites of passage like showers, baptisms, and funerals to help allay the anxiety. The specialists who deal in the implementation of these ceremonies command respect and are validated through their perceived power. They help to guide individuals through these difficult times. Midwives were such specialists. They had folk knowledge of birth and death. The death of a baby was especially traumatic, and because the midwife was the closest individual to the unbaptized soul of the newborn, she was often suspected of evil. Some people believed that she had the power to contract with the devil and sell him the souls of babies.

In this painting by Francisco Goya (1746–1828), midwives offer the souls of dead children to Satan, who has assumed the form of a goat.

> versation is like burning fire, and the Proverbs say that she takes possession of man's precious soul and the strongest men are ruined by her. And Ecclesiastes further says: "And I find more bitter than death the woman, whose heart is snares and nets, and her hands as bands." And others have said she is the vessel of the Devil. . . . In the second place, the Lord, who is all powerful, could have become incarnate as a man directly in some miraculous way, but he chose instead to dwell in the womb of a woman. . . .[22]

Theology loomed large, but so did superstition. In such an ambivalent universe, prayer was the answer and final authority reposed in the church. In a world without science, any unexplained phenomenon served as an example of punishment from God, and illness fell into this category. Augustine considered all human suffering as the "manifestations of innate evil, consequent upon original sin."[20] Tales of miraculous cures, often of tabloid-page intensity, were told and retold to generations of believers. Prayer, not people, could conquer disease. Typically during this era, monasteries were the centers of learning. The church alone had the time, the resources, and the technology to publish, but it showed no interest in medical and scientific knowledge. Religious orders selectively perpetuated only those data which fit in with their teachings. New information that questioned, contradicted, or expressed uncomplimentary ideas was quickly discarded. Moreover, Genesis provided the rationale for a clergy already enthusiastic to silence women as much as possible. In the words of Tertullian:

> You give birth, woman, in suffering and anguish. . . . And do you not know that you are Eve? She still lives in this world, as God's judgment on your sex. Live then, for you must, as an accused. The devil is in you. . . . You were the one who deceived man, whom the devil knew not how to vanquish.[24]

(Incidentally, it is puzzling why there is so much misogyny in Christianity, especially since Jesus himself did not articulate a negative attitude toward women. Nor did he appear to be fearful of menstrual pollution. The gospel according to Mark recounts the story of "a certain woman" who had had "an issue of blood twelve years and had suffered many things," and who came to Jesus for healing. "If I may touch but his clothes," she said, "I shall be whole." According to Mark's report, "And straightaway the fountain of her blood was dried up; and she felt in her body that she was healed of that plague.")[25]

At first, early medicine—an art more than a science—was not reconcilable with Christianity. Galen, who wrote "On the Anatomy of the Uterus," expelled Christian students as acolytes. The reason for this was simple: The Christian belief in divine healing was based on prayer to the new god, and for early Christians, Greek medicine was considered pagan and unwanted. But as Henry Sigerist observes, "When Christianity became the official religion of the Roman state it had to compromise with necessity by taking over the cultural heritage of the past. Christians became physicians and treated patients by applying the doctrines of pagan medical writers."[26] With one exception: Many "pagan" thinkers still diagnosed women's uterine problems as curable with sex. Paul of Aegina, for example, taught that "coitus was the best remedy for melancholy since it restored reason to those afflicted with mania [i.e., women]."[27] This was a thorn in the paw of early religious thinkers who felt sex was evil.

For now, suffice it to say that as a result of Augustine's anti-sex attitudes and misogyny, early Christianity acted to devalue women. In the philosophy of Augustine, sexual desire in men was equivalent to the sinful act itself, and women were to be blamed for men's lascivious thoughts. The church moved ruthlessly to suppress women, and any woman who dared to dress like a man, preach, or perform any role perceived as male was viewed as a deviant, thus a heretic. Women now had three strikes against them: the legacy of Eve's alleged seduction, their alleged power over nature, and the heresy they committed when they aspired to a leadership role in the church. Indeed, in the eyes of church fathers like Tertullian, women were the cause of all humanity's evil and suffering, and they would be paying their dues throughout eternity.

ENDNOTES

1. Tertullian, "De Cultu Feminarum." Quoted in George Seldes, *The Great Quotations: A Unique Anthology of the Wisdom of the Centuries* (New York: Carol Publishing Group, 1993), p. 680.

2. Arno Karlen, *Sexuality and Homosexuality: A New View* (New York: W. W. Norton & Company, 1971), p. 70.

3. Augustine, "Celiacus I." Quoted in Seldes, p. 71.

4. Uta Ranke-Heinemann, *Eunuchs for the Kingdom of Heaven* (New York: Penguin, 1990), p. 74.

5. Vern L. Bullough, Brenda Shelton, and Sarah Slavin, *The Subordinated Sex* (Athens: University of Georgia Press, 1988), p. 98.

6. Vern L. Bullough and Bonnie Bullough, *Sexual Attitudes: Myths and Realities* (Amherst, N.Y.: Prometheus Books, 1995), p. 22.

7. Ibid., p. 23.

8. Vern L. Bullough and Bonnie Bullough, *The Subordinate Sex: A History of Attitudes toward Women* (Urbana: University of Illinois Press, 1973), p. 118.

9. For a more comprehensive discussion of church attitudes toward women, see Bullough and Bullough, *The Subordinate Sex,* especially chapter 5, "Christianity, Sex, and Women."

10. Edward Shorter, *A History of Women's Bodies* (New York: Basic Books, 1982), p. 41.

11. Sibylle Harksen, *Women in the Middle Ages* (New York: Abner Schram/Universe Books, 1975), p. 37.

12. Jeffrey Burton Russell, *Witchcraft in the Middle Ages* (Ithaca: Cornell University Press, 1972), p. 79.

13. Harksen, p. 38.

14. Ibid.

15. Russell, p. 176.

16. Ibid., p. 79.

17. Sigrid Brauner, *Fearless Wives and Frightened Shrew* (Amherst: University of Massachusetts Press, 1992), p. 8.

18. Russell, p. 79.

19. Bullough and Bullough, p. 223.

20. Brauner, p. 9.

21. Vern L. Bullough and James Brundage, *Sexual Practices in the Medieval Church* (Amherst, N.Y.: Prometheus Books, 1982), p. 37.

22. Umberto Eco, *The Name of the Rose* (New York: Warner Books, 1984), p. 300.

23. Ilza Veith, *Hysteria: The History of Disease* (Chicago: University of Chicago Press, 1965), p. 49.

24. Quoted in Monique Alexander, "Early Christian Women." In *History of Women in the West, Volume 1: From Ancient Goddesses to Christian Saints,* Georges Duby and Michelle Perrot, eds. (Cambridge: Belknap Press, 1992), p. 409.

25. Mark: 5:25–29.

26. Henry Sigerist, *Civilization and Disease* (Chicago: University of Chicago Press, 1970), p. 140.

27. Bullough and Brundage, p. 16.

Chapter 3

The Medieval Uterus

It's a good thing that universities developed after monasteries. Perhaps some knowledge was lost in translation—from Greek to Arabic to Latin, ad infinitum—but it was better than having no medical information at all. According to Laurinda Dixon, "The medical school at Salerno adopted a gynecology based on Galenized Arabic theory, spiced with a sprinkling of Hippocrates and blended into a Christian matrix."[1] The work of Soranus of Ephesus, who had much earlier written that "the uterus falls forward, not because it is animal like, as some believe, but because, nearly resembling others parts, it has sensitiveness," had not yet been translated in its entirety.[2] Soranus's advice to women regarding virginity upheld and supported the cultural norms, but his reasons were far more practical. He had observed childbirth and saw its inherent dangers and the consequent morbidity and mortality that existed in a time without anesthesia or antibiotics.

As people who have lived with, and accepted, the medicalization of childbirth, we have no idea of the struggles that pregnant women endured a few thousand years ago. It is difficult to picture a situation where the head of an emerging newborn might be refused exit by a stubborn pubic symphysis, or a scenario in which a helpless husband and the extended family witness a labor that continues for more than five days. Even so, we know that the major cause of death for women was childbirth until fairly recently. It was a successful pelvis that admitted the moldable biparietal diameter of the newborn. Archival material written by Paul of Aegina describes the problems of the laboring uterus (see Appendix I).

Medieval drawings based on earlier writings describing the fetus in utero indicate that medieval physicians had not directly handled many dead pregnant women. The best-known work of Soranus, *On Diseases of Women,* had been translated into Latin and illustrated with drawings of the uterus that show imaginatively mature, straight-limbed, miniature adults, eyes open, dancing in anticipation of birth. His cat-headed uterus is certainly more accurate than the seven-chambered versions proposed by Galen and others (Figure 13), and some of the drawings reflect an understanding of podalic version and "turning" before birth. But, on the whole, medieval knowledge of the uterus was focused more on theological issues than anatomical ones, though the issues were related in important ways. The question "When does life begin?" was of interest, as well as "When does the soul enter the body?" St. Thomas Aquinas moved the time of entry forward from Aristotle's fortieth day for males and eightieth day for females to sometime between the fourth and fifth month, when quickening occurred. Interestingly, Aquinas saw no reason that females had to wait longer for their souls than males.[3] Much later in the nineteenth century, Pope Pius IX would settle these discrepancies, declaring that all souls entered at conception, therefore abortion at any time was a sin.

Illuminated manuscripts of the time that show caesarean sections are somewhat deceptive in representing the operation's success for the mothers of these infants. The apparently drastic

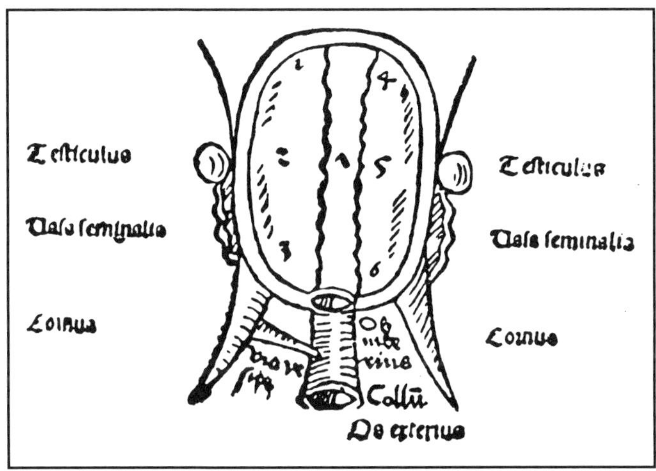

From Charles Singer, *A Short History of Anatomy from the Greeks to Harvey.* Reprinted by permission from Dover Publications, Inc.

***Figure 13.* The Uterus in 1501.** The seven-chambered uterus can be found in old anatomical drawings; in this version, the artist, M. Hundt, numbered each compartment. The belief was that males developed in the three right-hand chambers, females in the three left-hand chambers, and hermaphrodites in the middle one. (The Latin word for "left hand" is *sinestra,* which also meant "unfavorable." Its meaning has since come to include *sinester,* "evil.")

surgeries depicted were probably performed on dying or already dead women (Figure 14). Other medieval art on childbirth shows women attending other women. What is indisputably accurate in these pictures is the posture of the mother giving birth: She sat upright or was partially supported by other women, allowing gravity to aid her laboring uterus (Figure 15).

Although dissection was not totally forbidden, the ability of doctors to obtain human specimens was sporadic and depended on epidemics and criminal executions. Mondino de Luzzi (Mundinus of Padua) wrote his *Anothomia* in 1316, and though it was allegedly based on actual observation, he erred miserably when he described the uterus as divided into seven cells. Charles Singer attributes this error to Mondino's reliance on the writings of the "muddle-headed magician Michael the

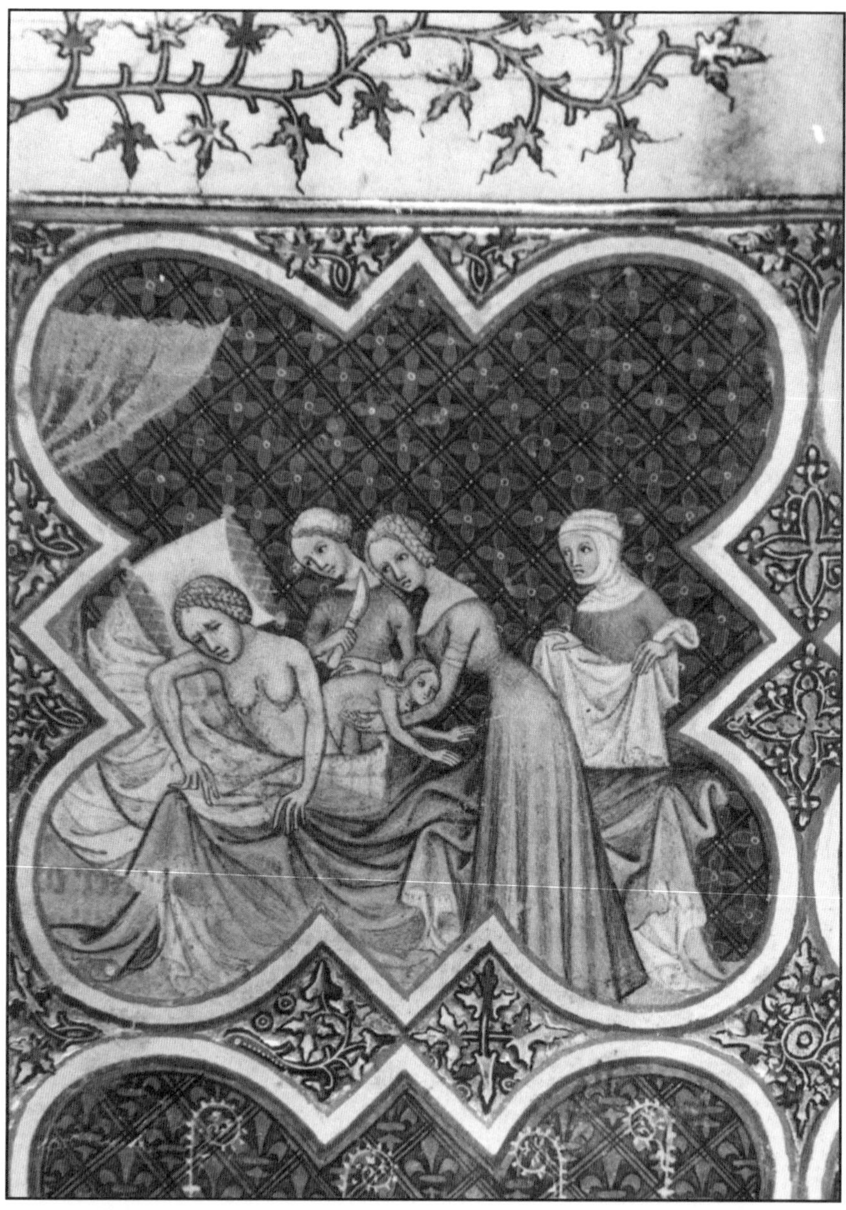

Jean Bondol. *Histoire ancienne jusqu'à César.* [Paris], c. 1375, vol. II, f. 199. Oslo/London: The Schøyen Collection, MS. 27.

***Figure 14.* A Medieval Caesarean Section.** The stress of labor and child-birth in a healthy woman is obvious, but when the baby is unable to get through the birth canal, there are two problems to confront: saving the life of the baby and saving the life of the mother. Soranus knew how to "turn" a baby in order to remove it vaginally as if it were dead, thus saving the mother's life. If the woman died prior to giving birth, removal via an incision in the abdomen was attempted. Many early medical sources report the use of caesarean sections. Albert Lyons and R. Joseph Petrucelli state that c-sections were performed in ancient India. Could this rather have been the mythical birth of Siddhartha, the baby boy formed from the union of a white elephant and the princess Maya? He was allegedly born from his mother's right side. Another myth, the birth of Asklepios, tells of his removal from his dead mother's abdomen by his father, Apollo. Numa Pompilius (715-673 B.C.E.) declared that if a woman died during pregnancy, her baby was to be cut out of her. A famous Roman general, Scipio Africans, is said to have been delivered by c-section, and the source of the word "caesarean" may have been his nickname (*caesar,* for "elephant"). However, most sources agree that the word was derived from Julius Caesar, who is supposed to have been born by caesarean section from his live mother, Aurelia. Although there are many artistic renderings of babies being born in this way, it is unlikely that the mother lived very long, presuming she survived the surgery.

In this medieval French image of 1375, a woman surgeon and two midwives are shown performing a caesarean section. It was not until after the Renaissance that literature describing the procedure was available. Much later—in the late nineteenth century—Max Sanger advocated using sutures to promote healing and proper suspension of the uterus. Later still—in the twentieth century—anesthesia and antibiotics allowed for safe surgery.

Scot" (Figure 16), whose works were based on Aristotle's *De Animalibus.*[4] Mondino also repeated many of Galen's errors, but the book he wrote became the standard, and would eventually go through forty editions.[5]

The notion of borrowing, translating, or copying a medical work for so long without actually testing its assertions may seem ridiculous to the modern reader, but in Europe before the thirteenth century, medical knowledge was severely restricted and obtained mainly through rote learning. As Vern and Bonnie Bullough point out,

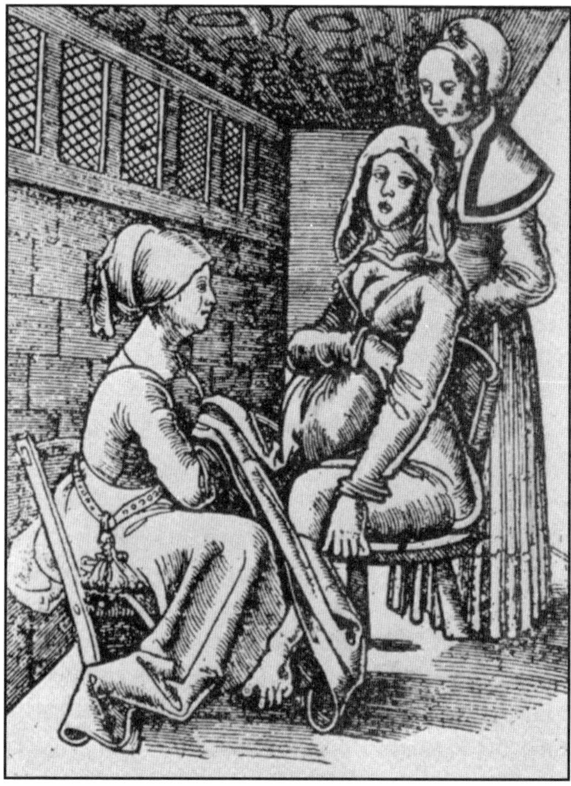

From the copy of the 1513 edition of the *Rosengarten* in the library of the Royal Society of Medicine. Reprinted with permission from Charles C. Thomas, Publisher, Ltd., Springfield, Illinois.

***Figure 15.* A Midwife-Attended Birth.** Midwives, not male physicians, attended women giving birth. The birth chair had no seat and was shaped like a horseshoe with legs and a back. The parturient woman sat upright to aid the downward pressure on her body during labor. One midwife sat facing her to observe and wait; she might have massaged the woman's labia and abdomen with oils or soothing emollients. Another midwife stood behind the woman and gave both moral and physical support. Feminist scholars believe that an entire pharmacopoeia of herbal analgesics were employed in labor and parturition by midwives. This tradition was lost, and all their knowledge made obsolete, by subsequent religious and medical prohibitions. Childbirth was an event in which knowledge between women was shared. A midwife was usually a woman who had personal experience of giving birth as well as a neighborly knowledge of the pregnant woman.

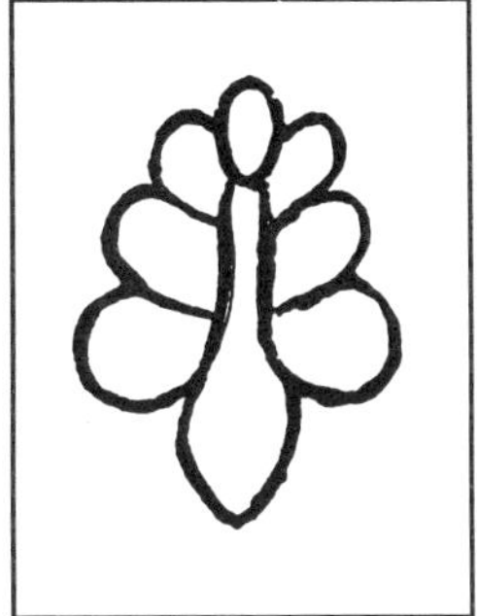

***Figure 16.* The Uterus of Michael Scot.** According to Charles Singer, the anatomists who drew a seven-chambered uterus were probably influenced by the writings of Michael the Scot (1178–1234). This seven-celled uterus is very different from the seven-chambered model seen in Figure 13 (Hundt's) and less accurate than the cat-headed uterus based on Soranus's descriptions (Figure 10). This example is a tracing of a fourteenth-century illustration of the uterus.

> During the early Middle Ages . . . much of the medical heritage of the Greeks was neglected by Western Europeans. It was rediscovered in the tenth, eleventh, and twelfth centuries through contacts with the Moslems, Jews, and Byzantine Greeks, and it was this rediscovery that gave rise to the medieval university and the powerful surgeons of the later period.[6]

In fact, the Deans and Masters of Medicine of the University of Paris held that "medicine was a science transmitted by texts, not a craft to be learned empirically." That's why Jacoba Felicie, a woman who practiced medicine in Paris, was prosecuted: She had "visited the sick, felt their pulses, examined their urine, bodies, limbs, prescribed drugs, collected fees and cured her patients."[7] According to William Minkowski,

> Faculty members were deeply offended by her use of what they viewed as techniques only for licensed doctors, such as examining urine by its physical appearance; touching the body; and prescribing potions, digestives, and laxatives. . . . The prosecution's entire case rested not on Felicie's proven incompetence but on her failure to be properly licensed by the university. . . . Not a single effort was made to test Felicie's knowledge and understanding of disease and its management. That she, as a woman, was ineligible to attend the university was ignored. . . . [S]he argued . . . for the right of wise

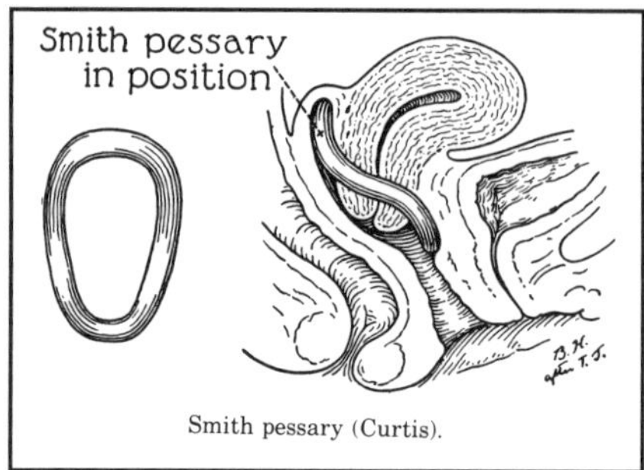

Dorland's Illustrated Medical Dictionary, 25th Edition (1974). Reprinted by permission of W. B. Saunders Company.

***Figure 17.* Pessary.** The pessary recommended by Trotula probably did not look like the Smith type pictured above. The word "pessary" comes from the Latin *pessarium,* an oval stone used in certain games. The device, however, was probably employed the same way a modern pessary is used—inserted in the vagina and retained to support and/or occlude the mouth of the uterus. Of course, if the woman was celibate, she could use the pessary to help keep her womb from wandering.

> and experienced—even if unlicensed—women to care for the sick. With even more spirit she asserted that it was improper for men to palpate the breasts and abdomens of women.[8]

Another female healer of the Middle Ages was the legendary Trotula (Trota), who taught at the University of Salerno. Was she a healer, a midwife, a learned and respected professor married to a male professor—or a myth? Texts disagree. In any event, *Practica secundum Trotam,* a text on women's diseases, as well as *Trotula Major* (*Ut de Curis*) and *Trotula Minor* (*Cum Autor*), two key obstetrical and gynecological texts of the time, are all attributed to her. In his book *An Introduction to the History of Medicine,* Fielding H. Garrison reviews the controversy:

> Malgaigne and Sudhoff show Trotula is not a person but the title of a book which asserts that Trotula was a nickname common to all Salernian midwives (*communiter Trotula vocata*). According to Daremberg and De Renzi, it is the name of an authoress, whom some supposed to have been of the Ruggiero family and the wife of the elder Platearius.[9]

Whatever the truth concerning their author, these treatises were sympathetic to the sad lot of women who did not have sex. *Ut de Curis* even recommended the use of a pessary (Figure 17), while *Cum Autor* diagnosed uterine fits as due to a superabundance of spoiled seed, an earlier Galenic idea.[10] The *English Trotula,* a translation into English of Trotula's work, contains complex and bizarre remedies, advice about conception, pregnancy, and childbirth, and methods guaranteed to cure "wind in the uterus" and other female problems.[11] Wind in the uterus, for example, was diagnosed by Trotula as the result of spoiled seed cooling and corrupting the blood: "From this superabundant and spoiled seed a certain cold substance is formed which ascends to certain parts which by common use are called 'collaterals' because they are neighbors to the heart, and lungs, and vocal organs, whence an impediment to the voice is wont to happen."[12]

Two other healers of the Middle Ages should also be mentioned here: Hildegard of Bingen and St. Walpurga. Hildegard caused controversy from the time she was young. When her parents were embarrassed by her visions and auditory hallucinations, they sent her away to a kind of boarding school. While there, Hildegard reached her maturity and, as a young woman, wrote her revelations, mainly texts on healing. She was probably the first ethnobotanist because she employed herbal remedies in her recommended therapies. Like most healers of the time, Hildegard depended heavily on the humoral theory but recognized mental states like "frenzy, insanity, obsession, and idiocy."[13] She also sympathized with the melancholy of nuns and recommended sapphire as an anti-aphrodisiac.

St. Walpurga did not suffer the indignities of Jacoba Felicie because she was a nun and therefore validated to take care of the sick. She used uroscopy (the examination of urine) without punishment, though uroscopy was not the clinical science we know now. The image of the healer holding a flask to the light belies its mystical epistemology: The intent of the examiner has more to do with the supernatural than with albumen content.

Despite the contributions of these women, authority was the

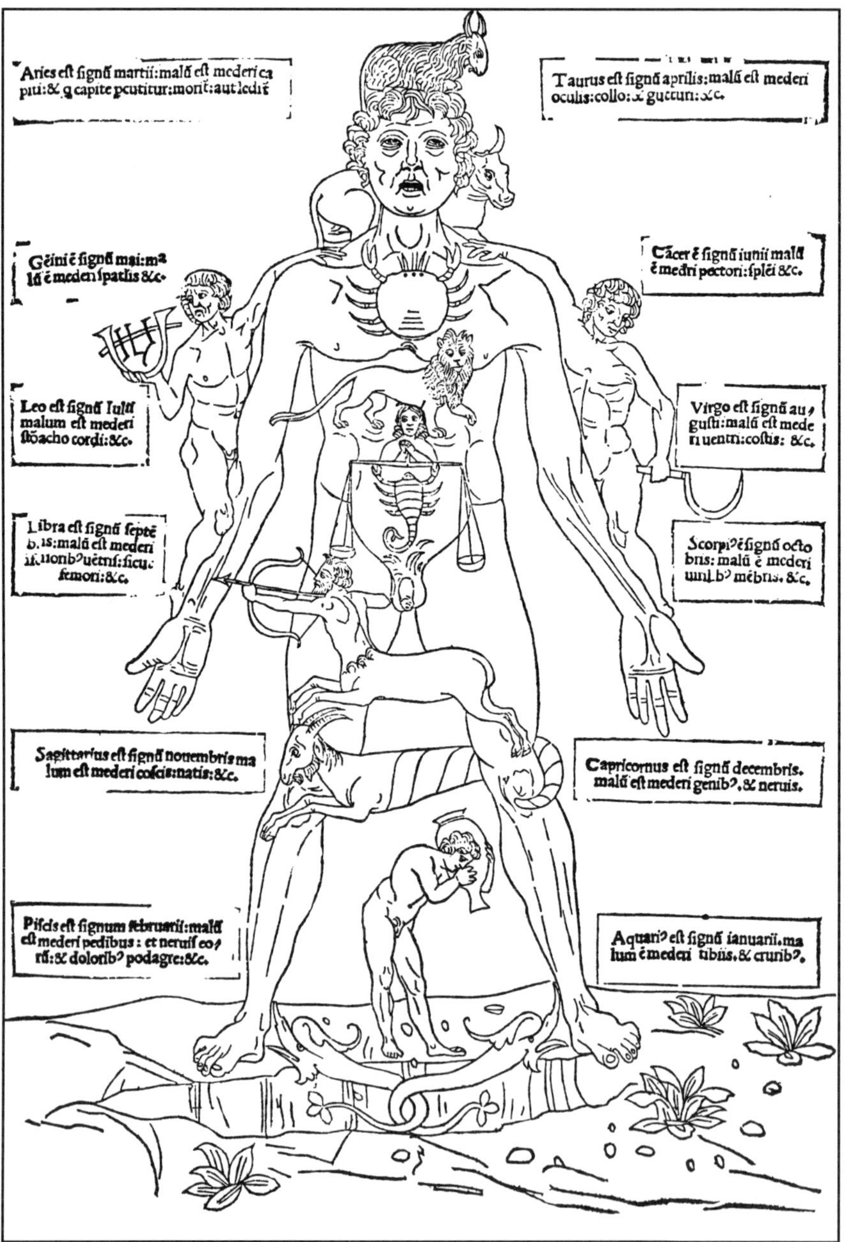

Reproduced from *Medicine and the Artist (Ars Medica)* by permission of the Philadelphia Museum of Art and Dover Publications, Inc., New York, N.Y.

***Figure 18.* Zodiac Man.** In the Middle Ages, anatomy, astrology, and humoral theory combined were thought to provide knowledge for healing. The paradigm of body parts and their associated zodiac signs gave rise to diagrams that barber-surgeons would use to predict the time of the year when bloodletting would be most effective. This fifteenth-century model from Ketham's *Fasciculus Medicinaei* depicts an obviously male model. Earlier French images (circa 1413 to 1416) depict an androgenous model centered in an eye-shaped world turned vertically, with each constellation shown alongside its corresponding month. March is at the top, September at the bottom, June and July to the left, and November and December to the right. Scorpio was associated with the organs of generation; using the zodiac paradigm, if a person had a problem in the pelvis, the best time to be bled was in the fall. Likewise, head trouble was optimally treated between Aries and Pisces or in March, according to the cosmos. Later, as knowledge about blood vessels became more sophisticated, the charts showed bleeding points without the zodiac signs or other supernatural references.

---

catch-word of these times and the (male) clergy was the final authority. Important medical texts like *Ut de Curis, De animalibus, De usu partium,* and Avicenna's *Canon* were endlessly recycled, each time rewritten before handing them down to the next reader. Sometimes a paragraph would contradict the paragraph immediately before it, but there were unspoken rules that did not allow texts to be questioned. Avicenna's *Canon* held that "the instrument of generation in woman is the womb (*matrix*) and that it was created to resemble the instrument of generation in man, namely, the penis and its accompanying parts." This kind of authority provided the impetus and the direction for various artists and physicians to render the uterus in the likeness of a penis. If Galen wrote that the uterus had seven compartments, it was because he did not want to differ with the church; in reality, he had only seen a pig's uterus and that had *three* chambers.

According to the seven-chambered model of the uterus, females were conceived in the left three compartments, males in the right three, and hermaphrodites in the middle one. Arabic texts were a little more realistic: They had a sac-like uterus with two tubes attached. In *The Practica Pantegni,* a work written by

Ali ibn al-Abbas al-Majusi and Constantine (the latter an African scholar who lived with Benedictine monks and translated Arabic works on Greek medicine), the authors wrote that the "inner wall of the uterus was lined with hairs whose purpose was to retain both sperm and fetus."[14] All women were assumed to have a bicornuate uterus like those of dogs, cats, and pigs: a two-tubed structure that could accommodate multiple embryos, attached to a long birth passage.

Another influential text of the period—this one from the Salerno school where Trotula taught—held that "the womb contained two orifices: the *collum matricis* . . . an external orifice through which coitus was accomplished, and the *os matrici*, an internal orifice."[15] The *Anatomia magistri Nicolai physici* proposed that there was a female vein "which funnel[ed] a portion of the menstrual blood into the womb and another portion into the mammary glands, there to be transformed into milk for the nourishment of the newborn."[16] Still other texts held that since woman was the inverse of man, her genitalia consisted of one tube and two testicles (ovaries). And in astrology—a different sphere of "learning," but one still incorporated in the belief system of healing—there was the "zodiac-man," a person more androgenous than male, drawn with the corresponding signs of the zodiac on his/her body as well as an assortment of symbols (Figure 18). These charts were used by barber-surgeons in their choice of the right time to bleed people.[17]

ENDNOTES

1. Laurinda Dixon, *Perilous Chastity* (Ithaca: Cornell University Press, 1995), p. 21.

2. Herbert Thoms, *Classical Contributions to Obstetrics and Gynecology* (Springfield: Charles C. Thomas, 1935), p. 4.

3. Vern L. Bullough and Bonnie Bullough, *Sexual Attitudes: Myths and Realities* (Amherst, N.Y.: Prometheus Books, 1995), p. 148.

4. Charles Singer, *A Short History of Anatomy from the Greeks to Harvey* (New York: Dover, 1957), p. 81.

5. Albert Lyons and R. Joseph Petrucelli, *Medicine: An Illustrated History* (New York: Harry N. Abrams, Inc., 1987), p. 331.

6. Vern L. Bullough and Bonnie Bullough, *The Emergence of Modern Nursing* (London: McMillan, 1969), p. 31.

7. Lois Magner, *A History of Medicine* (New York: Marcel Dekker, Inc., 1992), p. 110.

8. William Minkowski, "Women Healers of the Middle Ages: Selected Aspects of Their History." *American Journal of Public Health* 82, no. 2 (February 1992): 293.

9. Fielding H. Garrison, *An Introduction to the History of Medicine* (Philadelphia: W. B. Saunders Company, 1929), p. 150.

10. Dixon, p. 24.

11. Magner, p. 269.

12. Quoted in Vern L. Bullough, *Sex, Society and History* (New York: Science History Publications, 1976), p. 53.

13. Magner, p. 109.

14. Claude Thomasset, "The Nature of Woman." In *A History of Women in the West, Volume 2: Silences of the Middle Ages,* Georges Duby and Michelle Perrot, eds. (Cambridge, Belknap Press, 1992), p. 52.

15. Ibid., p. 53.

16. Ibid.

17. Brian P. Kennedy, "Artists and Anatomists." In *The Anatomy Lesson,* Brian P. Kennedy and Davis Coakley, eds. (Dublin: National Gallery of Ireland, 1992), p. 16.

CHAPTER 4

The Renaissance Uterus

As humanism uprooted theology during the Renaissance, knowledge was able to flower. The uterus, however, was still curiously depicted (Figure 19), and the mysteries of fertilization, pregnancy, and fetal growth were presented in equally enigmatic ways. Menstrual blood was still believed to be polluting to a woman and had the tendency to cause disease or "corrupt" if trapped inside her body.

Anatomical terms for certain parts of the uterus were based on male anatomy (testiculus, vasa seminalia) since woman's body was thought to be the inverse of man's. And since women had testes, female seed or semen was believed to be produced by those analogous organs. This concept was not new. Aristotle had denied the existence of female seed; only males had seed, according to him. But Hippocrates, who taught that mixing both male and female seed was necessary in order to form the embryo, believed that female semen was an essential part of the reproductive process. Taking it one step further, he also believed that women ejaculated totally, not partially, and that there were two

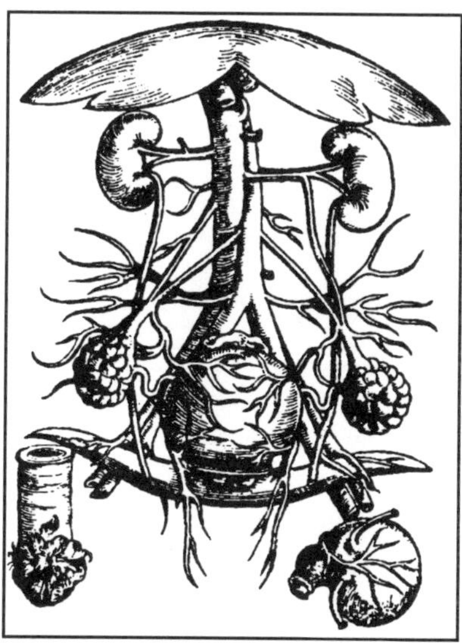

Courtesy of the National Library of Medicine, History of Medicine Division.

***Figure 19.* The Uterus in 1554.** Although men have traditionally described women's bodies, their documentation has not been too accurate. In this image from an obstetrical text by Jacques Rueff, the uterus is the phallic-appearing appendage suspended like a pod from a transverse structure.

kinds of female ejaculation: one inside the womb which made it moist, and the other outside the womb if it was open wider than usual.[1] Francisco de Valles (Franciscus Valesius) recognized the potential threat to gender hierarchy implicit in this idea: If both sexes had semen, then both would have power and females could conceive without intercourse.[2] To reassure his readers, de Valles quickly concluded that nothing could be more absurd: "One needs to reply that female semen, even though it has powers . . . yet is of less strength than that it might alone suffice for conception, for it is colder than the male variety."[3] But the power of spoiled female seed to do harm was still taken for granted: "It was generally believed that female seed shared with menstrual blood the tendency to corrupt and become noxious if, for some reason, trapped in the female body."[4] Another physician, Abraham Zacuto, wrote that " 'suppressed menses' and retained semen could deteriorate in the womb and turn so noxious as to equal the strongest poison."[5]

How were doctors to deal with this problem? In her book *Medical Ethics in the Renaissance,* Winfried Schleiner cites an anecdotal example from Peter Foreest in his book on women's diseases, *De Mulierum Morbis*:

> A widow, 44, . . . in May of 1546 was taken for dead and was lying unconscious, I was urgently called to her . . . it was a case of suffocation because of retained seed. The women present . . . were only making her worse. We also applied bindings to her hips, [because] by inflicting pain, [the binding] stirs matter downward and prevents the rising upward of vapors. Because of the urgency of the situation, we asked a midwife to come and apply ointment to the patient's genitals, rubbing them inside with her finger. And thus she was against hope brought back to consciousness. For such titillation with the finger is commended by all physicians . . . particularly for widows and persons abstaining like nuns—less so for younger and servant women or those who have a husband; for them a better remedy is to sleep with a man.[6]

Of course, this treatment raised ethical questions. Even Zacuto himself asked if a "God-fearing physician [could be] allowed to expel from the uterus the poisonous semen by titillation and friction of the genital area of women in mortal danger, deprived of all their senses and their breathing."[7] A physician by the name of Ranchin also asked the question "whether one is allowed to rub women or handle their parts in their hysterical paroxism," though he wiggled out of answering it definitively by saying that the use of this remedy should be left to the individual physician's conscience.[8] Ranchin went on to say,

> Those who approve do not lack authorities and arguments. First Galen puts forth the story of some widow restored to health by a midwife inserting her finger in her womb and thus evacuating her semen. From this grew the practice that most [women] use instruments skillfully hollowed out and similar in form to the male penis in order to provoke voluntary pollution

> and guard against hysterical symptoms. Secondly, Avicenna recommends that midwives insert a finger into the vulva and rub it diligently until the seminal material is expelled.[9]

Ranchin distinguished between sexual activity and friction as a cure for uterine problems and recommended the latter, although he felt such rubbing was "abominable and damnable particularly in virgins, since such pollution may spoil virginity." But other writers of the time defended this masturbatory-type therapy, stating that it was neither sinful nor criminal. The important element was the matter of volition: If patients shed the bad seed against their will or at least without their own consent, it was acceptable. The argument continued on into the seventeenth century: Moxius (1587–1612), in his book *De Methodo Medendi,* included a chapter entitled "Is the Physician Permitted to Expel Directly the Corrupt Semen that Induces Death?"

The world of images had parallel paradoxes. Renaissance artists tried to make their observations of both living and dead bodies consonant with written works but found troubling discrepancies. Their new freedom to explore and document the present exposed the ignorance of the past. The uterus that entered the Renaissance had seven chambers: three for males, three for females, and one for hermaphrodites. The uterus that left the Renaissance was a single vessel with only one chamber equally available to male and female embryos.

This shift was not comprehensive with regard to anatomic detail. Da Vinci learned and thus believed that, after conception, any retained menstrual products would travel to the breast to aid in the production of milk. He drew a uterus with vessels going directly to the breast. He also played it safe with respect to the many centuries of Galenic anatomy; his uterus is equivocal with respect to seven chambers. The paradigm that changed concerned *ways of seeing*. Da Vinci gave the world spectacularly detailed anatomical drawings and created a system that referenced the position of the observed in relation to the observer (*norma frontalis, norma lateralis, norma dorsalis, norma ventralis*)—an important concept in a time when realistic images were strictly forbidden, especially those that could reflect divine workings.[10] It is hard to imagine a world without graphics, but for many years physicians opposed the use of anatomical drawings because they felt images detracted from the text.[11] Other Renaissance artists followed da Vinci's lead. Jonathan Sawday argues that Berengarius's uterine images of 1522 "demonstrate the primacy of ocular evidence—the evidence of dissection—over classical (written) authority"[12] (Figure 20). But this particular image resembles external male genitalia and does not demonstrate any particular knowledge of internal female anatomy at all. The other uterus attributed to Berengarius (Figure 21) resembles the uterus of 1493 (Figure 22) with its horns and tubes leading to the breasts. Neither image is likely to convince the twentieth-century viewer that ocular evidence prevailed over classical authority.

Nevertheless, the growth of ideas in the Renaissance continued, traveling between countries by horseback and via the printing press. Cardinal Luis of Aragon was impressed with da Vinci's knowledge and related, "This gentleman has written of anatomy with such detail, showing by illustrations the limbs, muscles, nerves, veins, ligaments, intestines and whatever else there is to discuss in the bodies of men and women, in a way that has never yet been done by anyone else."[13]

Bolder than da Vinci was Andreas Vesalius, whose students dared to steal the freshly interred body of a monk's mistress, a woman who had mysteriously died of "strangulation of the uterus." Her uterus is so distorted that were it not for the caption in Book V of Vesalius's *De Humani Corporis Fabrica,* one would mistake it for a penis (Figure 23); the uterus appears phallic because the vulva and the vagina—which Vesalius calls the cervical canal—are included. Coincidentally, Vesalius published *De Humani Corporis Fabrica* the same year that Copernicus shocked the world with *De Revolutionibus Orbium Coelestium,* a book whose ideas were upheld by Galileo despite his near-execution for heresy. According to Sawday, " 'It is not

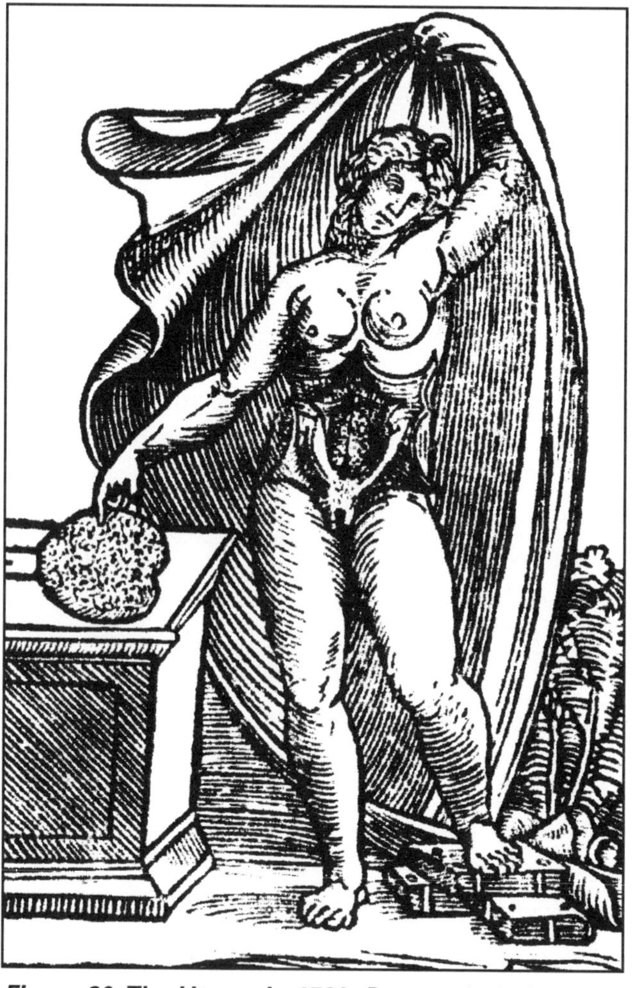

Image courtesy of the National Library of Medicine, History of Medicine division.

Figure 20. **The Uterus in 1522.** Berengarius's *Isagoge Breves* (also known as Berengario's *Isagoge Brevis*). In *The Body Emblazoned,* Jonathan Sawday quotes Thomas Laqueur: "The woman gestures toward the excised uterus which has been placed on the pedestal from which she herself has just stepped. . . . She demonstrates the primacy of ocular evidence—the evidence of dissection—over classical (written) authority." (This is symbolized by her foot on the books.) "The vigorous gesture with which she points to the uterus seems to demonstrate her mastery over that organ, an erstwhile independent agent of the body. . . . [But it could also mean] her identity is entirely determined by the uterus, to an extent that it is possible for her own position on the pedestal to be assumed by just one anatomical organ: the uterus, in effect, is the woman."

Image courtesy of the National Library of Medicine, History of Medicine division.

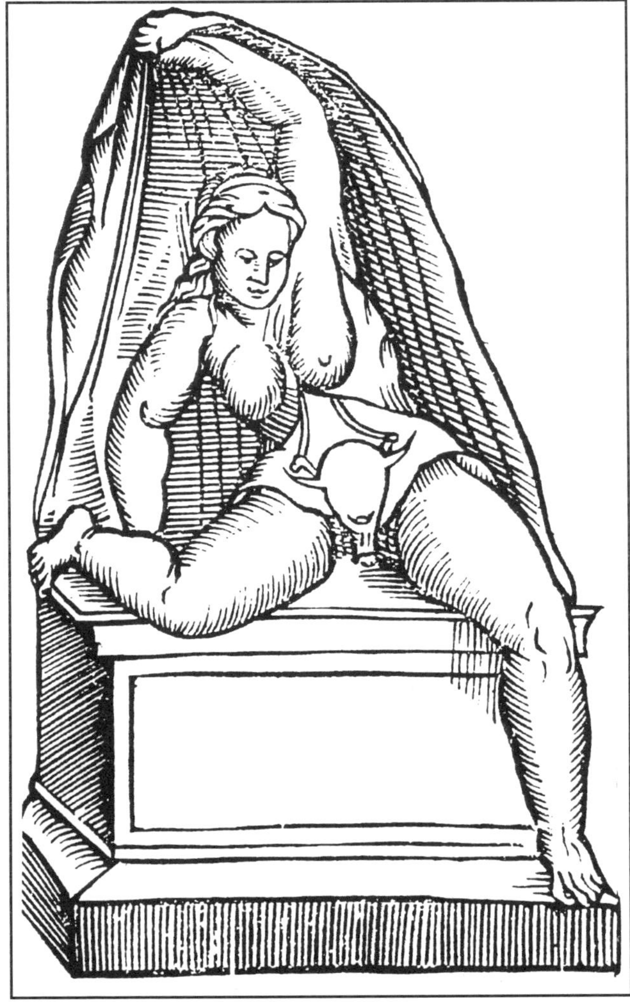

***Figure 21.* Another Uterus in 1522.** The woman in this picture is not yet a willing participant in her anatomical discoveries. She is the "seen," and as such displays her mysteries but does not take part in the revelation. Anatomical models, in addition to teaching medical students about the human body, were available for artists to sketch so their art would be more realistic. Although the uterus depicted here is also drawn by Berengarius, it has horns similar to those in the 1493 image by Ketham (see Figure 22). The tone of the picture is active rather than passive, vital rather than sorrowful.

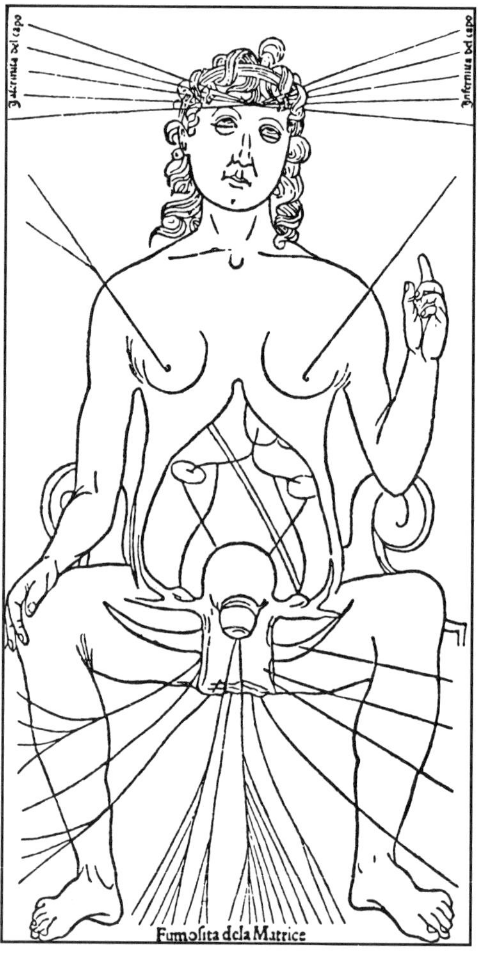

From Charles Singer, *A Short History of Anatomy from the Greeks to Harvey.* Reprinted with permission of Dover Publications, Inc.

***Figure 22.* The Uterus in 1493.** This woman and her uterus are taken from a work titled *Fasciculo di Medicina* (1493) by Ketham, an Italian transcription of Mondino's *Anothomia* (1315). The uterus is depicted with horns, and for good reason: During the course of his lecture, the anatomy professor would sit far from the body being dissected and read from a book that told where each organ was and how it should look. An assistant would perform the actual autopsy and hold up each part as the professor described it. When an organ differed from its description in the book, it was presumed to be anomalous or pathological—the exception rather than the rule. This uterus was the model for Berengarius; the difference is in their bodies, mainly in the passive versus active facial expression.

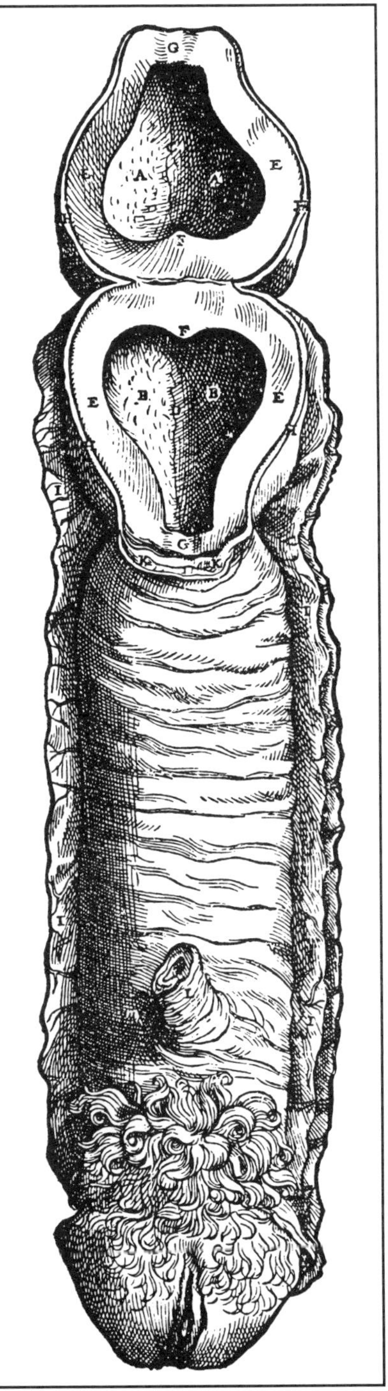

***Figure 23.* The Uterus of Vesalius.** This phallic uterus, part of the Fifth Book of Vesalius's *De Humani Corporis Fabrica,* circa 1543, is reportedly inaccurate because it was hastily removed from the dead body of a young woman who was the sex partner of a monk. In fact, her limbs were dismembered and her entire skin was flayed and removed in a frantic attempt to make her unrecognizable after her parents and the monk discovered that her body was missing from the tomb.

According to the story, Vesalius and his students were so desperate to examine a female body that, according to J. B. de C. M. Saunders and Charles D. O'Malley, they dug her up and quickly "encircle[d] the external genitalia with a knife, split the symphysis and excise[d] the vagina and uterus in one piece after severance of the urethra."

Whatever the story, one is struck by the profound persistence of the "woman is the inverse of man" worldview, even in someone as revered as Vesalius.

the sun,' the title page of the *Fabrica* insists, 'which lies at the centre of the known universe. The world is neither geocentric, nor heliocentric, but utocentric: the womb is our point of origin.' "[14] Sawday points out other parallels: "Both Copernican macrocosmic and Vesalian microcosmic theory rested not only on observation and calculation, but on an aesthetic derived in part from Horatian ideas of decorum and . . . Neoplatonic ideas of symmetry and order."[15] Both Da Vinci and Vesalius observed, but both failed to directly reproduce what they saw.

What Vesalius did that was new was to lecture and demonstrate at the same time. Mondino is the only other pre-Vesalian anatomist said to have taught this way. Prior to Mondino and Vesalius, clerics sat in a high chair far above the dissection table and recited from a text while a student labored below, cutting and holding up the organs he removed for public scrutiny. Neither student nor reader coordinated body part with written word, nor did they have the opportunity to work together regularly since each student needed an opportunity to dissect. Although Vesalius probably dissected only about twelve women, he keenly sought answers to questions about their generative organs. His first opportunity presented itself when the uncle of an eighteen-year-old girl asked him to verify the cause of her death. The uncle suspected that she had been poisoned; Vesalius hypothesized that, rather than murder as a cause of her death, inadequate pulmonary ventilation had led to pneumonia or pleurisy:

> From constriction of the thorax by a corset the girl had been accustomed to wear so that her waist might appear long and willowy, I judged that the complaint lay in a compression of the torso around the hypochondria and lungs. Although she had suffered from an ailment of the lungs, yet the astonishing compression of the organs in the hypochondria appeared to us to be the cause of her ailment, even though we found nothing that would indicate strangulation of the uterus except some swelling of the ovaries. After the attendant women had

> left . . . in company with the physician I dissected the girl's uterus for the sake of the hymen. The hymen, however, was not entirely whole but had not quite disappeared, as I have found is usually the case in female cadavers, in which one can barely find the place where it had been. It looked as if the girl had ripped the hymen with her fingers either for some frivolous reason or according to Rhaze's prescription against strangulation of the uterus without the intervention of a man.[16]

Thus Vesalius observed that strangulation could occur without a uterine etiology, although in some of his other writings he uses the phrase "uterine strangulation" as though he accepted its clinical reality. Another uterus that Vesalius examined was from a female criminal who had been executed. She had tried to delay her gallows date with the excuse that she was pregnant, but the judge ordered midwives to present their opinion and they disagreed with her claim. This woman's body, shown without arms, legs, or a head and represented lying on the ground, has been immortalized as Figure 24 in Book V:

> The present figure has been drawn for the special purpose of showing the position of the uterus and bladder just as they occurred in this woman and without our disturbing the uterus in any way. None of the uterine membranes has been destroyed, but everything is seen intact just as it appears to the dissector immediately upon moving the intestine to one side in a moderately fat woman.[17]

On the matter of lactation, Vesalius, like his predecessors, believed that pregnancy diverted blood that would have become menstrual blood to large superior blood vessels leading to the breast, which then converted it to milk. Despite his errors, however, Vesalius's influence was profound. The old theological paradigms of the body were no longer valid and Vesalius became the giant upon whose shoulders Paré, Sylvius, Fallopius, Eustacius, Columbo, Harvey, and Servetus were to stand.

Late Renaissance anatomical drawings also reflected this

change. The facial expressions on the women shown are quite different from the earlier pained and sorrowful representations. There are now elaborate and inviting background scenes, with flowers or landscaped gardens. Indeed, woman's body is now represented as "the divine workmanship of God."[18] Another difference was between "seer" and "seen": Art was yet one more way that men were able to look at women's bodies. Jonathan Sawday points out that "the female subjects of the Renaissance anatomical dissection were represented as willing participants in the complete process."[19] As we shall see, the aesthetic enhancement of these bodies is still more pronounced in the seventeenth century, where woman's gravid body is displayed like a plant with layers of leaves that, when unfolded, reveal a fetus attached to the placenta with an umbilical cord. Although the woman depicted appears unfazed by her eviscerated condition, the dead tree stump with a couple of slender offshoots behind her symbolizes the presence of death (Figure 24).

Another important Renaissance text, *Der Swangern Frawen und Hebammen Rosengarten,* was written in 1513 by Eucharius Rösslin. The *Rosengarten* was a compendium of all the knowledge that Rösslin could cull from midwives, although he degraded them in his introduction:

> I'm talking about the midwives all,
> Whose heads are empty as a hall,
> And through their dreadful negligence
> Cause babies' deaths devoid of sense
> So thus we see far and about
> Official murder, there's no doubt.[20]

This work was written in the German vernacular so midwives could read it; later it was translated into Latin. The uterus is depicted as spacious by the artist, Erhardt Schoen, and the fetus is likened to a fully developed youngster. One well-known illustration shows a woman in a birthing chair, supported under her arms by a female attendant and facing the woman

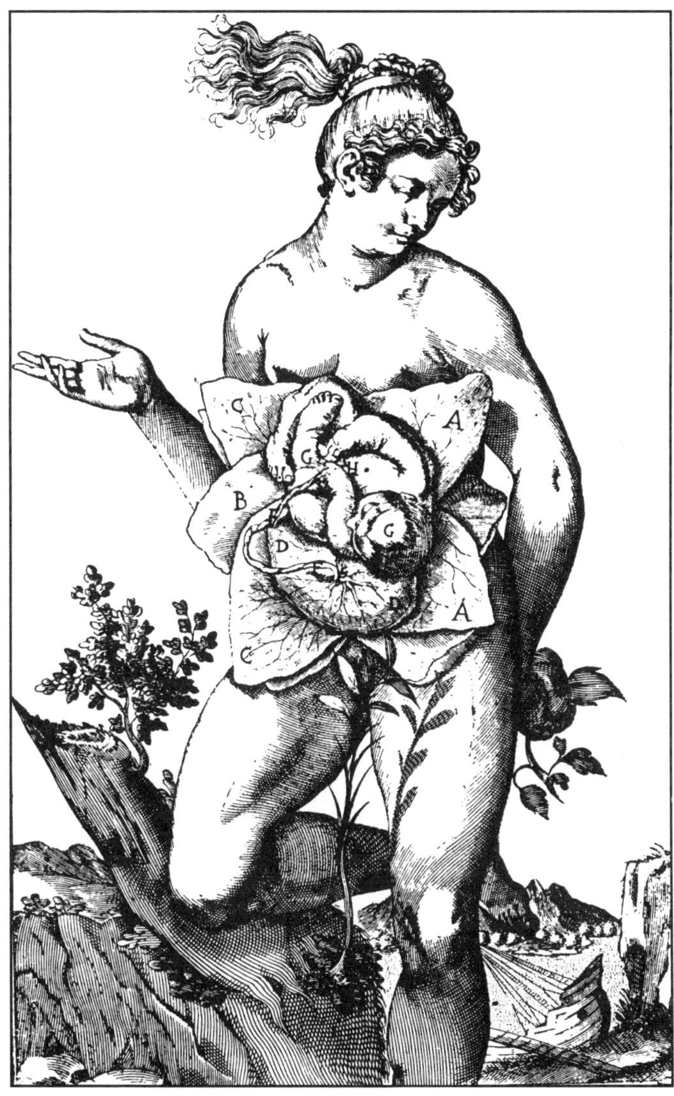

From Charles Singer, *A Short History of Anatomy from the Greeks to Harvey.* Reprinted with permission of Dover Publications, Inc.

***Figure 24.* Spigelius's Uterus of 1622.** In the seventeenth century, anatomical drawings of the uterus and the women who owned them showed a new realism. In the image shown here, the umbilical cord is attached to the placenta and the fetal posture and position are accurate. The relationship between birth and death is communicated by the dead tree trunk sprouting new buds aimed in the direction of the woman's pelvis.

who will deliver the baby. She wears no shoes and holds tightly to the bottom of the chair with her left hand. Her breasts are exposed and she looks away from the older woman, who sits on a stool facing her. Her facial expression is blunted, perhaps affected by an analgesic (see Figure 15). According to Herbert Thoms in his *Classical Contributions to Obstetrics and Gynecology,* Rösslin's book "was the first work dealing with obstetrics apart from medicine and surgery and, in its illustrations, gave for the first time printed figures of the birth chair, the lying-in chamber, and the positions of the fetus in utero. Some of the plates are of high artistic merit and were copied by subsequent writers."[21]

Midwives continued to play an important role throughout the Renaissance. Each European country had a midwife system, and although there was some variation on the theme, midwives were basically self-governing. In Baden, Switzerland, for example, an official midwife was recognized.[22] In Germany, there was an independent corps of midwives that can be traced back to 1298.[23] In other parts of Germany, a midwife corps was headed by a voluntary *obfrau* and no one had control over her. As Edward Shorter reports, "Under her control would be a handful of female midwife inspectors who were available if the salaried town midwives ran into emergencies. In order to become a midwife, there were only a limited number of positions and sometimes women waited more than ten years for an opening. They would be apprenticed and paid partially or fully by the city."[24] According to Hebbamerstan Heberling, "The first formal midwife oath . . . dates from Regensburg in 1452. It made the midwives promise to deliver all women, whether rich or poor, except for Jews; to bring any woman they may find doing deliveries unlawfully in front of the female board of supervisors; not to drink too much; and not to leave one woman in labor in order to deliver another who can pay more."[25] In Aachen, an additional requirement was that the midwife report all "secret births," and a 1544 ordinance in the town of Hildensen instructed midwives to pray repeatedly if a delivery were delayed.[26]

No matter how difficult the labor, midwives were expected

and required to aid in the delivery of healthy, viable, and undeformed fetuses. Moreover, midwives had very specific rules governing their profession. Some rules prohibited them from becoming educated at a university. In some rural areas, their social status was lowly and they were paid with goods rather than money. Perceived as a "necessary evil" in some communities and a necessary good in others, they were a class of women with varying statuses, depending on the degree of urbanization or contact with changing values.

In addition to physicians and village bureaucrats, the Church had an interest in midwives. In the tradition of the early Church, women were supposed neither to speak nor to teach, nor were they permitted to "tell men what to do." But because the practice of delivering children required some voice, midwives had at least a modicum of power. Indeed, to protect the souls of newborns who might not live, midwives were given the power to baptize, according to a church synod circa 1310.[27]

Throughout the fifteenth and sixteenth centuries, the laws governing midwives increased. Up to this point, male physicians had not been particularly interested in the problems of parturient women because modesty on the part of women, and embarrassment on the part of men, prevented male-attended childbirth in all but the most traumatic cases. This attitude is reflected in the English translation of the *Rosengarten,* which was published in 1540 with a new title, *The Byrth of Mankynde,* as well as the following disclaimer:

> Many think it is not . . . fitting in such matters to be intreated of so plainly in our . . . vulgar language, to the dishonour(e) of woman hood, and the derision of their own secrets by the detection and discovering whereof men it reading shall be moved thereby . . . every boy and knave reading them as openly as the tales of Robin Hood.[28]

Despite such sentiments, the possibility of professional medical assistance in childbirth was increasingly recognized. By 1554, another midwifery text was published in Switzerland, *Trostbüchle* by Jacob Rüff, which argued for the application of (male) medical knowledge to childbirth management. And educated male doctors had the political power to examine midwife candidates and supervise those in practice.[29] In England at about the same time, for example, a physician by the name of Andrew Boorde "proposed that every midwife be presented to the Bishop upon recommendation of 'honest women' who were prepared to testify that she was 'a sadde woman wise and discrete, having experience, and worthy to have ye office' . . . [and] beginning with Edmund Bonner, Bishop of London . . . the episcopacy began to license midwives."[30]

Inevitably, as men crept forward to dominate the birthing room, midwives were less needed; they were also more likely to be publicly accused as persons suspected of witchcraft or sorcery. Prejudged guilty, midwives were required to swear not to use sorcery or incantation and to baptize only with plain water. As Jane Donegan reports,

> Church inspectors were to inquire whether the practicing midwives in the region had been examined and licensed by the bishop. They were to determine if any of the women employed "witchcraft, charms, sorcery, or invocations," and to learn of cases in which the midwives, assistants or patients had exhibited signs of "disorder or evil behaviour."[31]

The gradual change from female to male midwives was now underway. Many pregnant women were not happy with the change. They feared horrible scenarios if men were allowed to attend births, and in most cases the men were not allowed to look. A drape placed around the man's neck kept his head in full view of others in the birthing room, a sort of monitor on his demeanor. This ritual of "not looking" was to last for hundreds of years, each century redefining the proper behavior for a male examining a female.

Interestingly, those very prohibitions against a male doctor looking at a woman's body were reversed when it came to examining women for signs of witchcraft. For a naked woman to be forced to expose herself to the scrutiny of a roomful of unfamiliar males was in itself an overwhelmingly frightening experience. As Anne Llewellyn Barstow observes in her book on the European witch hunts:

> It appears that jailers, prickers, [and] executioners . . . all could take their sadistic pleasure with female prisoners. And so could respectable ministers and judges. . . . These men took advantage of positions of authority . . . thus revealing that they wanted more from witch hunting than the conviction of witches: namely, unchallengeable sexual power over women. . . . In the witch hunts, the policy of forcing a witch's confession may have been a cover for making a socially approved assault on her body.[32]

Also in the Renaissance, a powerful document known as the *Malleus Maleficarum* or the *Hammer of Witches* was written by two churchy "experts" on witchcraft, James (Jacob) Sprenger, who later became the General Inquisitor for Germany, and Henry Kramer, a Dominican. Although it was published in 1483, the *Hammer of Witches* did not strike with its full force until nearly 150 years after its original publication, when it was translated into French, Dutch, English, and Spanish. All throughout Europe, women were hanged, drowned, tortured, and burned according to the rules of the *Malleus* (Figure 25). This holocaust of European women prosecuted and persecuted for witchcraft extended to the New World. Native American healers were murdered in both North and South America in the name of a Christian God, and as E. William Monter informs us, "In the English colonies about 40 people were executed for witchcraft between 1650 and 1710, half of them in the famous Salem Witch Trials of 1692."[33]

As the Renaissance drew to a close, the uterus was accorded one chamber, two tubes, and a generally phallic appearance. Though woman was no longer quite the mistake of nature or imperfection she had once been, she was still "a prisoner of the

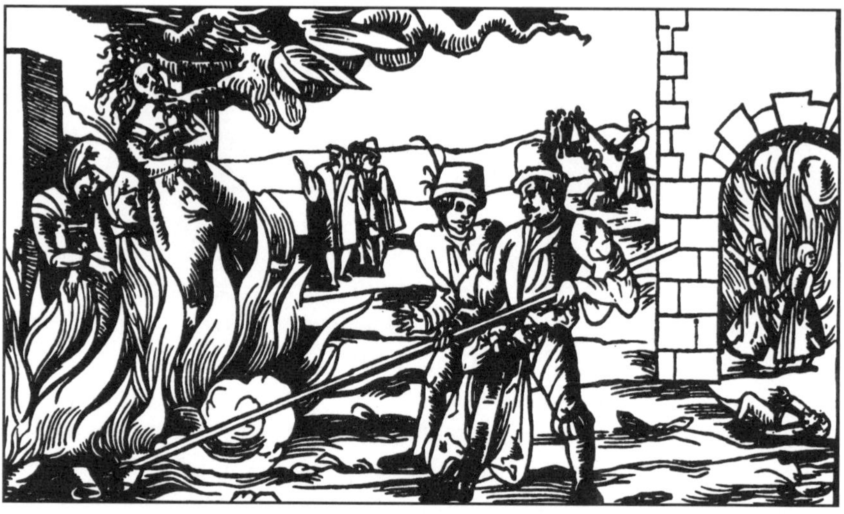

Courtesy of Dover Pictorial Archive Series.

***Figure 25.* Witches Burned at the Stake.** As Anne Llewellyn Barstow observes in her book *Witchcraze: A New History of the European Witch Hunts,* "Public tortures and executions of witches officially conveyed strong messages about the expectations and limitations of women in society."

strange organ that dwelled within her."[34] And the influence of the uterus on personality was still emphatically voiced, for example in the writings of Rabelais, the French satirist and physician (1494–1553), who wrote:

> [I]n a secret and intestinal place, a certain animal or member which is not in man, in which are engendered, frequently, certain humours, brackish, nitrous, voracious, acrid, mordant, shooting, and bitterly tickling, by the painful prickling and wriggling of which—for this member is extremely nervous and sensitive—the entire feminine body is shaken, all the senses ravished, all the passions carried to a point of repletion, and all through thrown into confusion. To such a degree that, if Nature had not rouged their foreheads with a tint of shame, you would see them running the streets like mad women . . . and this, for the reason that this terrible animal I am telling you about is so very intimately associated with all the principal parts of the body, as anatomy teaches us.[35]

In such a world, it's understandable that a term like "uterine furies" was considered diagnostic.

ENDNOTES

1. Winfried Schleiner, *Medical Ethics in the Renaissance* (Washington, D.C.: Georgetown University Press, 1995), p. 108.
2. Ibid.
3. Ibid.
4. Ibid., p. 111.
5. Ibid.
6. Ibid., p. 113.
7. Abraham Zacuto, *De praxi medica libri tres.* Quoted in Schleiner, p. 118.
8. Schleiner, p. 119.
9. Ibid., p. 120.
10. Robert Wallace, *The World of Leonardo* (New York: Time Incorporated, 1966), p. 105.
11. Ibid., p. 105.
12. Jonathan Sawday, *The Body Emblazoned* (London: Routledge, 1995), p. 215.
13. Edward Maccurdy, *The Notebooks of Leonardo da Vinci* (New York: George Braziller, 1956), p. 12.
14. Sawday, p. 71.
15. Ibid.
16. Charles D. O'Malley, *Andreas Vesalius of Brussels* (Berkeley: University of California Press, 1965), p. 63.
17. J. B. deC. M. Saunders and Charles D. O'Malley, *The Illustrations from the Works of Andreas Vesalius of Brussels* (New York: Dover, 1973), p. 170. Most people attribute anatomical drawings such as the skeleton pondering a skull to Vesalius, but the wood blocks were designed and drawn by Jan Van Kalkar and others instructed by Vesalius to illustrate his findings. The original six plates (*Tabulae Sex*) were modifications of his earlier "fugitive sheets" made for uneducated barber-surgeons and bath attendants. These templates carved in wood were intended for physicians and students because Vesalius wanted to make certain that each student would have accurate, not poorly copied, information.
18. Sawday, p. 23.
19. Sawday, p. 216.
20. Quoted in Edward Shorter, *A History of Women's Bodies* (New York: Basic Books, 1982), p. 36.

21. Herbert Thoms, *Classical Contributions to Obstetrics and Gynecology* (Springfield, Ill.: Charles C. Thomas, 1935), p. 52.

22. Shorter, p. 38.

23. Ibid., p. 37.

24. Ibid.

25. Quoted in ibid., p. 41.

26. Ibid., p. 41.

27. Ibid.

28. Thomas Raynalde, *The Byrth of Mankynde, Otherwise Named the Womans Booke.* Quoted in Jane B. Donegan, *Women and Men Midwives* (Westport, Conn.: Greenwood Press, 1978), p. 23.

29. Shorter, p. 41.

30. Donegan, p. 11.

31. Ibid.

32. Anne Llewellyn Barstow, *Witchcraze: A New History of the European Witch Hunts* (New York: Pandora, 1994), p. 132.

33. E. William Monter, "Witchcraft." In the *Grolier MultiMedia Encyclopedia* (Version 7.0, 1995).

34. Evelyne Berriot-Salvadore, "The Discourse of Medicine and Science." In *A History of Women in the West, Volume 3: Renaissance and Enlightenment Paradoxes,* Georges Duby and Michelle Perrot, eds. (Cambridge: Belknap Press, 1993), p. 358.

35. François Rabelais, *Tiers Livres.* Quoted in Vern L. Bullough and Bonnie Bullough, *The Subordinate Sex* (Urbana: University of Illinois, 1973), p. 192.

CHAPTER 5

The Baroque Uterus

How can it be that the seventeenth century is considered the Age of Reason when there was still so much superstition and violence, including the continued persecution of alleged witches? Perhaps it was the *modes* of examining knowledge rather than its *content* that were rational. Even so, now that the structure of the human body and the universe seemed comprehensible, it is odd that seventeenth-century scientists and philosophers did not readily challenge or expose many of the still-untested beliefs regarding women. It appears that the hungry mouth of the womb, integral to the prevailing concepts of women and their appetites, was not to be denied.

Anatomy determined destiny, biologically and socially. In her book *The Compleat Midwife's Companion,* Jane Sharp wrote that "what the woman provided was a place for the uterus to reside where it received the offerings of both male and female: the womb is that field of nature into which the seed of man and woman is cast, and it hath also an attractive faculty to draw in

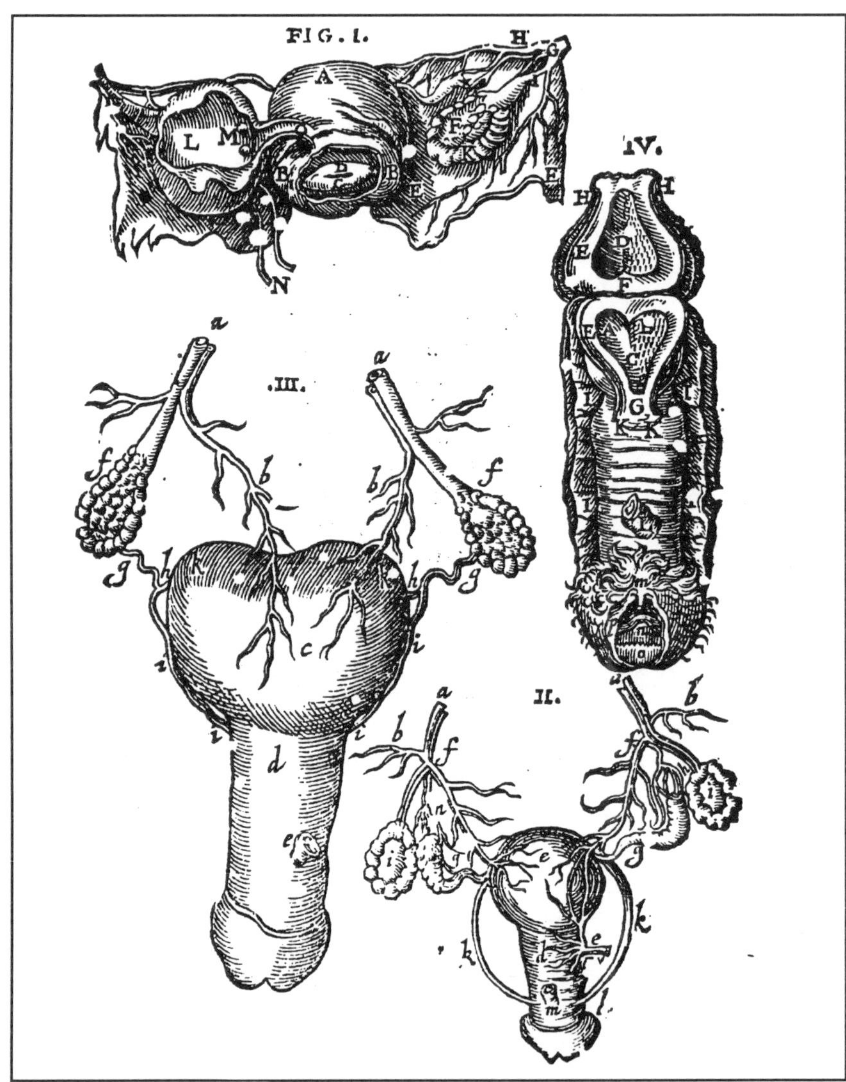

Figure 26. **The Uterus According to Ambroise Paré.** In this rendering by Thomas Johnson (1634), based on the over one-hundred-year-old gynecological writings of Ambroise Paré, the womb appears as an inverted scrotum attached to a phallic vagina, however "underdeveloped and imperfect." Note the similarity of Vesalius's uterus to the figure on the upper right. Humoral theory was still an important influence in the seventeenth century, hence the cure for the "uterine furies"—which afflicted nuns, widows, and "ancient maids"—was to sit in cold water and cool the overheated uterus, thus restoring the balance of humors.

a magnetic quality as the lodestone draweth iron, or fire the light of the candle."[1] But a shift in the ideological construct of that anatomy had occurred, as some artists now depicted women in more realistic and human terms. Earlier thinkers had posited woman's reproductive apparatus as mirroring man's, the inverse or reverse. It was common knowledge that, when exposed to cold weather, a man's testes would shrivel, moving inward and closer toward the body. Humoral theory taught that women were cold and moist, and so were female genitalia. That's why the uterus was to remain inside—women just did not have enough heat. Prior to Vesalius, and even a little after, women were perceived to be lesser, incomplete models of men. But woman's status was growing a bit; she would not remain solely a receptacle for the developing fetus too much longer.

Importantly, the Baroque period was to redefine the female body as an entity unto itself, not a poor imitation of man's. This may not be evident in the work of Ambroise Paré (Figure 26), but how much could Paré know about women? Granted, he did have a civilian practice in Paris, but most of his work was on the battlefield, treating gunshot wounds. And although he did write about obstetrics in his second book, his eyes observed the uterus through the filter of earlier anatomical paradigms. Paré is problematic not only because he believed the female body to be incomplete or defective, but also because of his peculiar renderings of serpents and other creatures he claimed to have seen inside the womb (Figure 27). He wrote an apocryphal history of a woman who gave birth to twenty babies in the course of two pregnancies. Paré also persisted in the interpretation of menstrual blood as a superfluous humor discharged because the female body did not have enough heat, the characteristic of a cold, moist temperament.[2] According to this theory, although the female body formed blood from nutritional intake, it did not heat it up enough to be useful. Menstruation was understood to be a symptom of dysfunction, proof that something was wrong with the female body. Woman's body was unstable because of her uterus, thus her total being was labeled erratic and insatiable.

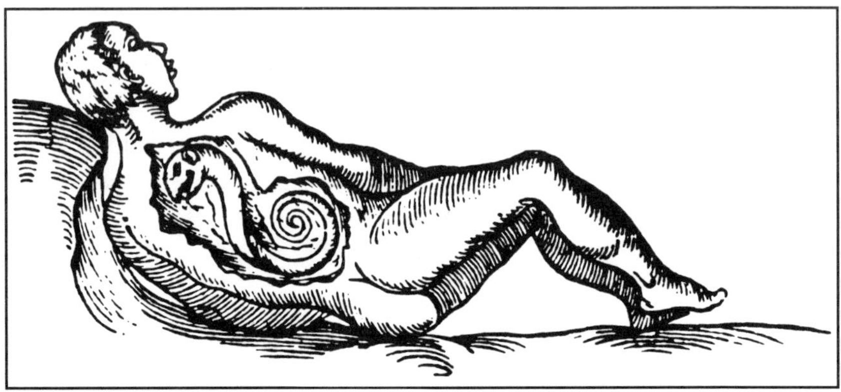

***Figure 27.* The Persistence of Myth.** Ambroise Paré was a cultural hero in the sixteenth century. Born in 1510, he rescued the study and practice of surgery from the barber-surgeons and traveling charlatans. In fact, Paré studied under the barber-surgeons but eventually surpassed his teachers. His first test came on the battlefield when Paré improvised a new treatment for gunshot wounds. Traditionally, the treatment for gunshot wounds was to apply boiling oil. Since Paré had none, he chose to apply salve. His patients fared better than those who had the oil treatment. His treatise on the subject, written in 1545, became a classic for wound treatment.

His knowledge of women and obstetrics, however, did not measure up to his wartime achievements. His study on *Women Who Have Given Birth to Many Children* told of a woman named Dorothea, who allegedly bore twenty children in only two pregnancies. His second book was written about childbirth and pregnancy; like Pliny, he witnessed many fantastic and surreal creatures residing in the womb, including the coiled serpent pictured here.

Paré also studied the anatomy Vesalius taught and incorporated it into his anatomy book. Despite anatomical experimentation, his rhetoric echoed anachronistic attitudes such as "woman is the inverse of man." Paré maintained that the uterus could be irritated by the behaviors and feelings of others as well as calmed by things it liked. (In other words, it had an identity.) He also held that menstruation was the discharge of superfluous blood that the cold, moist female body would not or could not use.

This changeable, unpredictable association with nature, reproduction, and abnormal propensity for sex explains why women, not men, were accused of witchcraft. Other reasons link fertility and sexuality and the control of both. According to historian Merry Wiesner:

> Many historians see social and economic changes . . . instrumental in the rise of witch trials. Europe entered a period of dramatic inflation during the sixteenth century and continued to be subject to periodic famines resulting from bad harvests; increases in witch accusations generally took place during periods of dearth and destruction caused by religious wars. . . . There was also a larger number of women unattached to a man, and therefore more suspect in the eyes of their neighbors.[3]

The peculiar focus on fertility, sexuality, and witchcraft has been explained by Carol Karlsen as one way a changing society dealt with the new economic power that women—particularly single women and widows—had acquired with personal property and real estate.[4]

The first major witch hunt occurred in Switzerland in 1427, but until there was a way for the *Malleus Maleficarum* to be more widely produced and distributed, its influence remained relatively local.[5] Once the printing press emerged, however, this codified, comprehensive tool for identifying witches insured that proper diagnosis, procedure, and outcome was available throughout most of Europe. According to the *Malleus,* the dangers posed by witches were legion. They could seduce men and take them away from their wives, they could cause crops to fail, and most importantly, they could make men impotent and unable to reproduce—and that really went against religion. As most European countries became obsessed with witches and witch hunting, midwives fell under particular suspicion.

Linguistically, *matrix* (another word for *uterus*) means "mother." The womb was "the receptacle in which 'a small creature of God' was formed . . . the most necessary and noble organ . . . in which the feminine quiddity resided."[6] And the midwife was inevitably the first member of society to see and handle the newborn. Should a deformed baby emerge, the midwife was required to identify the cause of that anomaly. Did God do it? Disease, as evidenced by the plagues in the Old Testament, was often a punishment decreed by God. Or was it the work of a witch? Only the midwife could say for sure. Then, too, midwives were required to record each birth with the name of the father—and in the case of an unmarried woman who was parturient, it was up to the midwife to document the name of the father. Not surprisingly, when the mother was unable to remember the name or even the act, it often turned out to be the work of the devil. Indeed, the close association of midwives with newborn babies and newborn souls put them in a precarious position as the witch hunts continued.

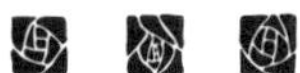

One brave physician ventured to refute the "evidence" of witchcraft in a scientific manner. According to Edward Jorden, since the uterus defined woman's total existence including her health, those fearful signs of disorder were physical, not supernatural. As he wrote in 1603:

> The passive condition of womankind is subject unto more diseases and of other sortes and natures than men are; and especially in regarde of that part from whence this disease which we speake of doth arise. For as it hath more varietie of offices belonging unto it then other partes of the bodie have, and accordingly is supplied from other partes with whatsoever it hath need of for those uses; so it must needes thereby be subject unto more infirmities than other parts are.[7]

Jorden believed that the uterus caused disease by two modes, one toxic and the other compressive. Such ideas were nothing new, and consistent with the themes of pollution and womb-wandering put forth by centuries of his forebears. The argument he used was that the symptoms which others attributed to witchcraft were in reality symptoms of the illness known to the ancients as "suffocation of the mother." He argued his case in an article entitled "A Briefe Discourse of a Disease Called the Suffocation of the Mother," written and dedicated to the president and fellows of the College of Physicians in London, "wherin [he] declared that divers strange actions and passions of the body . . . imputed to the Devil, have their true natural causes and do accompanie this disease." In a well-known court case of the time, Mary Glover, a fourteen-year-old girl, accused her neighbor, Elizabeth Jackson, of cursing and wishing her so much evil that she was afflicted with fits, pains, convulsions, and "venemous blasts." Jorden set forth to dispute that either "bloud or seed, offending in quantitie or qualitie, could probablie be accused in Marie Glovers miserie," citing Hippocratic dogma as his proof (i.e., "That nature in her first addresses to womanhood, should be so much surprized with a sudden over ruling adversarie . . ."). He then went on to explain that women are subject to many strange passions through the deprivation of two humors.[8] Unfortunately, Mary had not achieved menarche at the time of her first fit. Jorden had to expand his definition of "suffocation of the mother" to include "perturbations of the minde," and Elizabeth Jackson went to prison and the pillory.[9]

Anatomical drawings of the uterus and women's bodies produced during the seventeenth century demonstrate a more accurate understanding of internal organs. In addition, the display of the body was gaining public acceptance—so much so that ornate theaters for dissections were constructed to accommodate groups of spectators as well as doctors and artists studying the body (Figure 28). Dead women were drawn in life-like poses, displaying their internal organs, sometimes even holding open their abdominal walls to display their reproductive organs. Drawings by Spigelius in particular represent the culmination of beauty in his depiction of graceful female bodies (though with masculine shoulders and limbs) revealing the secrets of reproduction (see Figure 24).

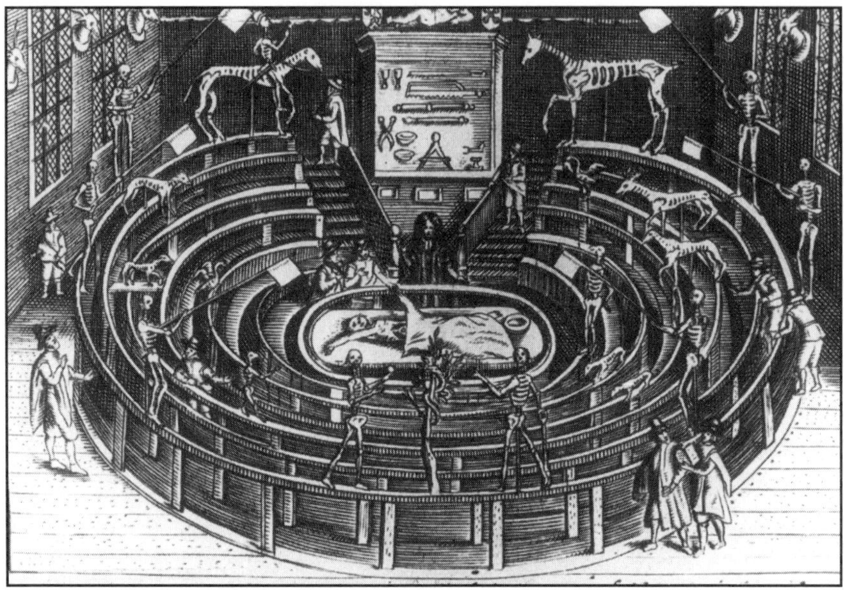

Photo courtesy of Anatomy Department, Leiden University.

***Figure 28.* Operating Theater in Leiden.** Operating theaters served as reminders to people of the fragility of life. In addition to being a sort of entertainment, dissections provided a clear-cut way of demonstrating the various causes of death. As science progressed in the direction of real as opposed to mystical explanations of "dis-ease," the worldview changed accordingly. The human and animal skeletons erected in various parts of the theater carried little flags bearing admonitions and sayings about morality and the fragility of life.

Although male anatomists displayed the female body in death, female midwives still tended the female body in life. Soon these two disciplines would meet. Not surprisingly, despite the increase in dissections, no uterus was found above the pelvic cavity. Lo and behold, it seemed the womb was stationary! Thomas Willis, who performed many autopsies, found that in all the women he dissected, the uterus lay within the pelvic basin, beneath the diaphragm. However, this fact did not deter some doctors from continuing to blame the uterus for unrelated medical problems. Indeed, throughout the seventeenth century and despite increasing evidence, those physicians who proposed other explanations for hysteria were still in the minority. "Perhaps it's a mind-body imbalance," stated Thomas Sydenham, the most renowned surgeon of the century, in *Of the Small-Pox and Hysteric Diseases.*[10] Nonetheless, his peers continued to stick to the wandering-womb model; as far as they were concerned, the only new paradigm was one that agreed with the old. As a result, the century abounded in hysterical diseases. Thomas Sydenham, staunch in his belief that hardly a woman existed who was free from hysteria, later found that men, too, could suffer from this malady. (He accordingly revised his thoughts on its etiology, attributing it to "disordered animal spirits.")[11] In the main, however, it was women—bedeviled, as always, by their uterus—who were most sorely afflicted. Women who had not yet married suffered from *de passione hysterica, de suffocatione uterina, de nymphomania, de febre virginum amatoria, de hysteromania,* and *de morbo virgineo.* Nuns suffered from *furor uterinus* and widows, appropriately, from "widow's melancholy" (see Appendix II). A new illness called *lovesickness* affected women who were abstinent or melancholy. Similar still was "the vapors," defined as "a morbid condition . . . caused by . . . depression of spirits, hypochondria, hysteria, or other nervous disorders."[12] (It was also called *hysteria passio.*) And an entire genre of Dutch painting revealed the "uterine furies," *chlorosis,* or "the mother-choking symptoms."[13]

Laurinda Dixon has written a book analyzing these "sickroom paintings." Her thesis is that the lovesick upper-middle-class women depicted in Flemish paintings are not really physically ill but are suffering instead from a culture-bound syndrome (Figure 29). She points out that the well-dressed and well-cared-for women are a little bit too healthy-looking to be truly ill; that they are merely acting out an expectation on the part of their society that they swoon or lose their faculties as a result of their preoccupation with a male lover. Earlier critics

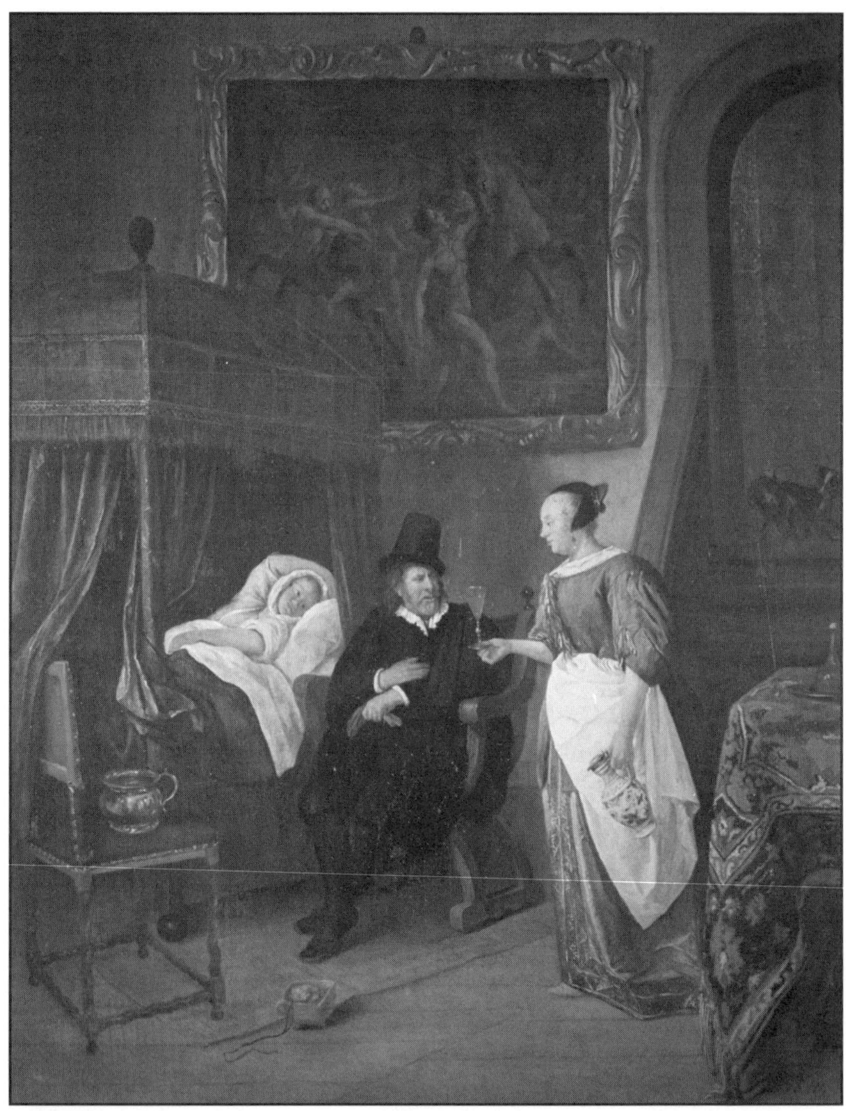

Jan Steen (1626–1679). *The Doctor's Visit.* Mauritshuis, The Hague, The Netherlands. Courtesy Scala/Art Resource, New York.

Figure 29. **Seventeenth-Century Dutch Sickroom Painting.** An entire genre of art focused on the uterus of the seventeenth-century woman and its dysfunction in various maladies, such as the "uterine furies." In this work by Jan Steen, entitled *The Doctor's Visit,* a sick girl suffers from a uterine disorder. One interpretation of this painting is that the erotic scene above her bed provides a clue to the young woman's problem. A burning string can be seen in one of the pots at the foot of her bed—a cultural survival from ancient times, when it was believed that fragrant fumes could be used to lure the uterus back to its rightful place.

---

hypothesized that these were pregnant women, fainting from morning sickness or disappointment that their partner had not married them. Dixon finds three major elements in the paintings. First, there is usually an erotic message in the background, in the form of a cupid or an amorous statue or painting. Second, there is usually an attractive young physician hovering intently over the woman, to whom she has exposed a bared breast. And third, there is usually an older woman in the background ready to burn a string or some other substance. This substance, when burned, will repel the uterus from its offending place and send it back to the pelvis, recalling the ancient Egyptian remedy.[14]

Although most medical care for women continued to be delivered by midwives throughout the seventeenth century, occasionally a surgeon would have to be called for difficult cases that might require exceptional physical strength because of the podalic version, breech, or problematic labor due to a constricted pelvis. A relationship did exist between female caregivers and medical men, albeit sometimes a grudging one. When an obstetrical manual, *La Commare Oriccoglitrice,* was published in Venice (Figure 30), it contained such clauses as "if she has suffered malpractice at the hands of some imprudent midwife," indicating a certain level of competitive misogynism.[15] Midwives felt that their virtues were gentleness, patience, and a history of shared experience; in denigrating midwives, male physicians stressed timeliness and efficiency. Since most men had never participated in the birth of a child, it was most likely their inexperience that accounted for their derogatory words;

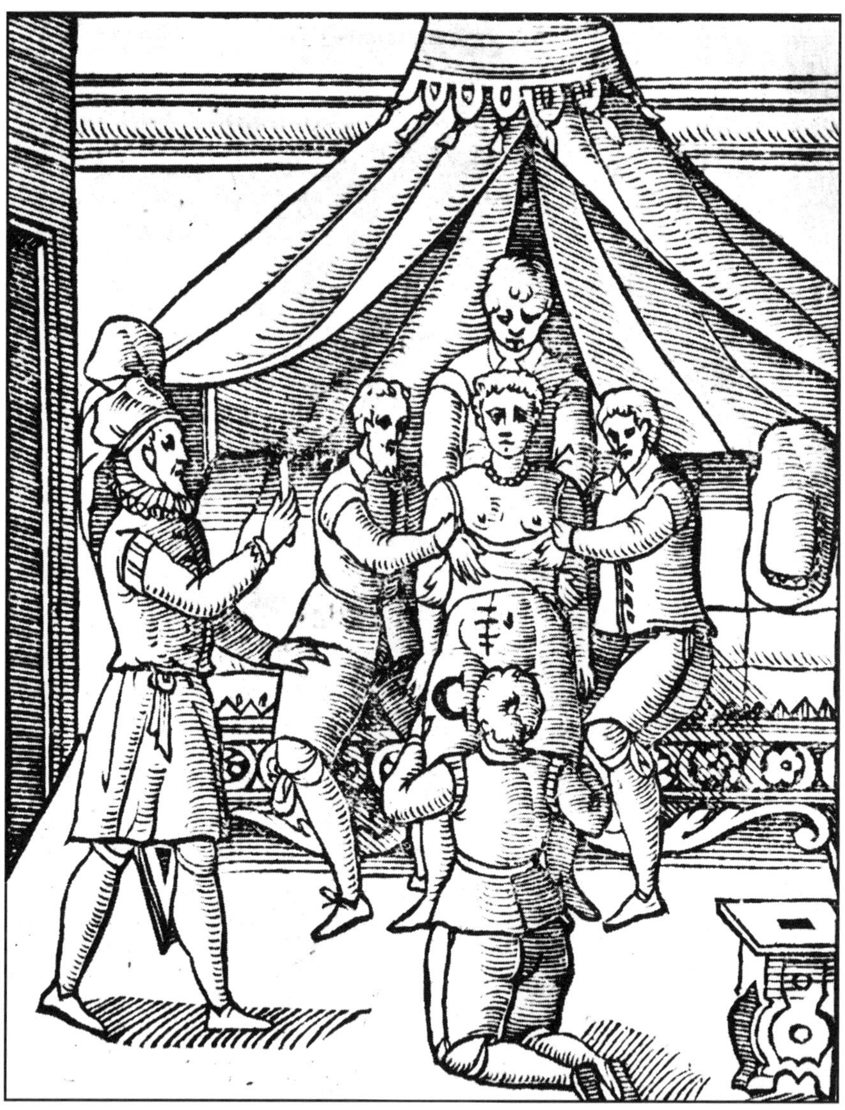

Photo courtesy of National Library of Medicine, History of Medicine division.

Figure 30. **How to Perform a Caesarean Section.** Scipione Mercurio (1540–1616) was educated in theology but later quit the monastery for medicine. He performed many dissections on pregnant women. His work *La Commare Oriccoglitrice* addressed normal childbirth, abnormal presentations, and the aftercare of mother and child. He is said to have introduced the caesarean section to Italy. Mercurio himself cautioned that not every surgeon was qualified to do caesareans, and recommended two positions for the procedure, including the one illustrated here: "When the patient's body has been cared for, the surgeon may choose two positions to be occupied by the patient; one, if she is strong and courageous; the other, if she is weak or afraid. If she is strong, let her be propped up so that she sits upon the edge of the bed in this way. . . ." He stipulated the need for six assistants, three to hold the woman and three for himself. In the section on marking and cutting the incision, Mercurio refers to himself as *Signore Iddio* ("Mr. God").

historically excluded from the birthing room, they just didn't understand the parameters of "normality." Of course, the attitude of surgeons toward themselves was quite different. The surgeon Scipione Mercurio (1540–1616), who is said to have introduced the caesarean section to Italy, was known to refer to himself as *Signore Iddio* ("Mr. God").[16]

Caesarean sections were one way that seventeenth-century doctors incorporated new techniques among their skills; forceps deliveries were another. Peter Chamberlen the Elder, a barber-surgeon, belonged to the Huguenot family that allegedly invented the forceps.[17] Along with his brother, Peter Chamberlen the Younger, he wanted to organize the midwives of England into a corporation (an association of professionals that acted as a regulatory body) and also to give them formal instruction in anatomy and the use of forceps. King James I was petitioned for his permission but referred the question to the College of Physicians, which eventually rejected the idea. A son, Peter Chamberlen III, again approached the College of Physicians but was rebuffed in his generation. Ironically, the midwives themselves did not want to be incorporated, even though they occasionally sought assistance from the Chamberlens and knew about forceps. They did not feel they would benefit from being incorporated. In fact, they had more knowledge with respect to normal births because of their traditional experience, the best teacher. Training for midwifery required day-to-day observation of both the work and behavior of skillful midwives, and they did not use instruments, nor did they want to.[18] According to Jane Donegan, the midwives also rejected Chamberlen's offer of anatomy lessons because "the English law that made felons available for anatomical dissections exempted gravid women," and it was pregnant women that they obviously had an interest in. Donegan also writes that the Chamberlen family kept the design of the forceps "a closely guarded family secret . . . advertising that they could deliver women in tedious and difficult cases. . . . Hugh Chamberlen, Junior, having no male heir to succeed him, let the general design of the family instrument be known before his death in 1728."[19] As with many inventions, the actual origin of the forceps is not consistent in all sources; independent use had already been documented by Smellie and Giffard. What is indisputable is that the technology of forceps use did change how the uterus would be controlled after the eighteenth century. By promoting forceps as the new technology that every woman would want in order to lessen her time in childbirth, male doctors had triumphed over nature—or so, at least, they advertised they had. In any event, women—especially upper-class women—demanded forceps-assisted deliveries, and their husbands were willing to pay for this high-tech advance in medicine (Figure 31).

In the early eighteenth century, obstetrical forceps helped establish male medical control of the uterus. Interestingly, now that the womb was known to stay fixed in the pelvis, hysteria started to wander up toward the brain, and its associations became less uterine and more psychological.

ENDNOTES

1. Jane Sharp, *The Compleat Midwife's Companion.* Quoted in Jonathan Sawday, *The Body Emblazoned* (London: Routledge, 1995), p. 215.

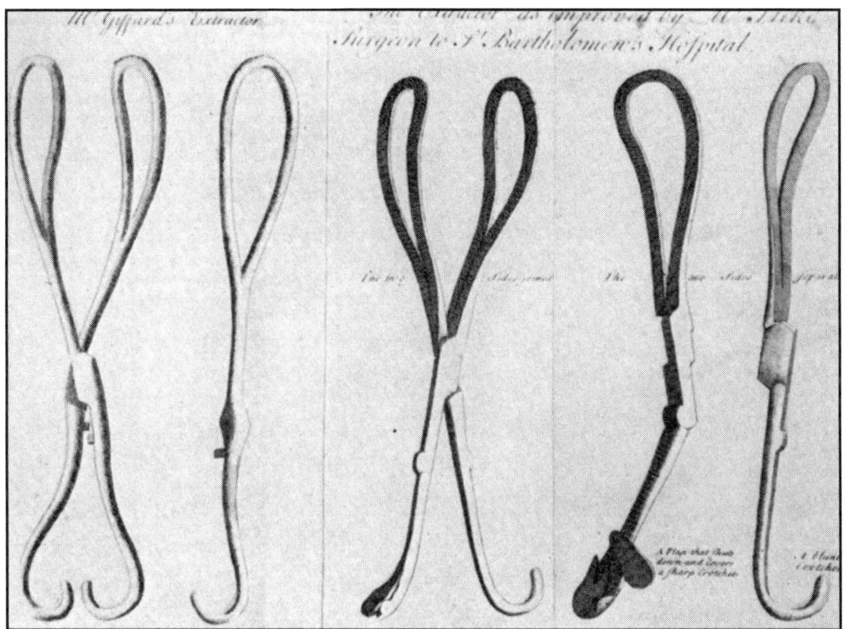

From Herbert Thoms, M.D., *Classical Contributions to Obstetrics and Gynecology*, 1935. Courtesy of Charles C. Thomas Publisher, Ltd., Springfield, Illinois.

***Figure 31.* Giffard's Extractors.** Although many texts credit the Chamberlen family with the first use of obstetrical forceps, others such as William Giffard, William Smellie, and Andre Levret are known to have employed them as well. William Giffard, a man midwife, kept records of his patients and in particular recorded the deliveries of two hundred and twenty-five women who had difficult presentations. His tome *Cases in Midwifery* was published posthumously in 1734. Giffard's other contribution was a technique to be used when the placenta separated from the uterus prematurely. According to H. G. Partridge, "Giffard was the altruistic and honorable physician who should receive full credit for introducing the forceps into common use in England." (Quoted in Herbert Thoms's *Classical Contributions to Obstetrics and Gynecology*.)

---

2. Evelyne Berriot-Salvadore, "The Discourse of Medicine and Science." In *A History of Women in the West, Volume 3: Renaissance and Enlightenment Paradoxes* (Cambridge: Belknap Press, 1993).

3. Merry Weisner, *Women and Gender in Early Europe* (Cambridge: Cambridge University Press, 1993).

4. Carol Karlsen, *The Devil in the Shape of a Woman* (New York: W. W. Norton, 1987), pp. xi–xv.

5. "Witchcraft," *Grolier MultiMedia Encyclopedia* (Version 7.0, 1995).

6. Berriot-Salvadore, p. 358.

7. Edward Jorden, "A Disease Called Suffocation of the Mother." Quoted in Philip Slavney, *Perspectives on Hysteria* (Baltimore: Johns Hopkins University Press, 1990), p. 16.

8. Michael Macdonald, *Witchcraft and Hysteria in Elizabethan London: Edward Jorden and the Mary Glover Case* (New York: Tavistock/Routledge, 1991), p. 96.

9. Ibid.

10. Quoted in Laurinda Dixon, *Perilous Chastity* (Ithaca: Cornell University Press, 1995), p. 52.

11. Lois Magner, *A History of Medicine* (New York: Marcel Dekker, Inc., 1992), p. 222.

12. Jane Mills, *Womanwords* (New York: Henry Holt & Company, 1989), p. 124.

13. Ibid.

14. Dixon, pp. 1–10.

15. Herbert Thoms, *Classical Contributions to Obstetrics and Gynecology* (Springfield, Ill.: Charles C. Thomas, 1935), p. 109.

16. Ibid., p. 110.

17. Jean Donnison, *Midwives and Medical Men* (London: Heinemann, 1977), p. 13.

18. Jane B. Donegan, *Women and Men Midwives* (Westport, Conn.: Greenwood Press, 1978), pp. 26–27.

19. Ibid., pp. 49–50.

CHAPTER 6
The Enlightenment Uterus

In the eighteenth century, microscopy, embryology, and dissection dealt a death blow to the humoral theory. Philosophers such as Voltaire, Kant, Rousseau, Diderot, and Montesquieu helped to fuel the renewed interest in rationality and its application to medicine and social problems. As Richard M. Brace points out in *The Making of the Modern World,* "it seemed altogether logical that if the workings of the physical universe could be shown to conform to laws . . . through the instrumentality of reason, the same methods could be applied with equal success to the workings of society."[1] And if women could be studied with the same techniques that revealed the secrets of the universe, the place of the female sex in the natural world would become evident. But this new rationality only served to bolster the set of definitions that upheld women's physical and mental inferiority and to reinforce the social stereotypes regarding them. Voltaire, for example, felt that "woman is weaker than man on account of her physiology."[2] His supporting evidence was that menstruation enfeebled her or caused illness if suppressed. Immanuel Kant dabbled in anthropology enough to contribute that women were more difficult to analyze than men and that the weakness of women was a vehicle to manipulate men. (Obviously, he didn't have *that* much trouble with analysis.) Granted, women were endowed with reason, but its quality was more concrete and less abstract than men's.[3] Good-looking women did not have reason at all: "Reason is never found . . . amoung those with beauty," said Montesquieu.[4] The great champion of human rights, Jean-Jacques Rousseau, regarded women as man-pleasers who were not entitled to receive equal pleasure in the male-female relationship. He wrote in *Émile,*

> Woman was made specifically to please man; if the latter must please her in turn, it is a less direct necessity. . . . If woman is formed to please and to live in subjection, she must render herself agreeable to man instead of provoking his wrath; her strength lies in her charms.[5]

From this it can be seen that eighteenth-century laws of nature were anything but enlightened for women. Rousseau went on to describe the proper behavior for women—silent, subservient, and secondary:

> A clever woman is a scourge to her husband, to her children, to her friends, to her servants, in short to everyone....Even if she possessed real abilities, it would only debase her to display them. Her honour consists in being unknown, her glory in the esteem of her husband, her pleasure in the happiness of her family.[6]

Sex (in the erotic sense) defined the nature of women, but not of men. It was nature which made her that way; according to Montesquieu, women were driven by an insatiable sexual appetite so powerful that men were forced to find ways to control their behavior for their own protection.

Despite these retrograde notions, a great curtain was drawn open during the Enlightenment to reveal the theater of the human body, displayed in whole or in parts, to be studied and used for teaching purposes. Even the church denied that it had ever prohibited dissection; the Bull of 1300, it explained, was merely against limb detachment and bone boiling. To compensate for this hiatus in learning, the Church displayed an unusual enthusiasm in its attitude toward biological knowledge, going so far as to donate the bodies of deceased ecclesiastics to be anatomized. The act of performing a post mortem was no longer exclusively pejorative: Once the fate of dead criminals, dissection was now an honor, an academic adventure, a way to share knowledge about how the human biological interior world affected the exterior world and vice versa. In Leiden, Hermann Boerhaave and Siegfried Albinus collected specimens from dissections, later housing the collection in a museum for students to study, and the operating theater at the Rijkuniversiteit was open for any interested spectators. Boerhaave described the Enlightenment physician's practice and mission as follows:

> He silently takes in the lessons from dissected bodies . . . he builds for himself a clear idea of the human frame. To this he adds a knowledge of the vital fluids; and tests it in the living person and his excretions by the aids of anatomy, chemistry, hydrostatics, and even of the microscope . . . he opens and explores the bodies of those whose maladies he has noted; . . . he groups together all the results of diseases and of remedies he has tried . . . he obtains a certain grasp of the history and the cure in each disease.[7]

Animal anatomy was now a model for certain processes or tests rather than representative of human structure. Inevitably, the growing interest in and need for human bodies led to the creation of a unique relationship between medical schools and grave robbers; respectable professors paid for fresh corpses, and a new class of crimes—bootlegging bodies—was born. Public

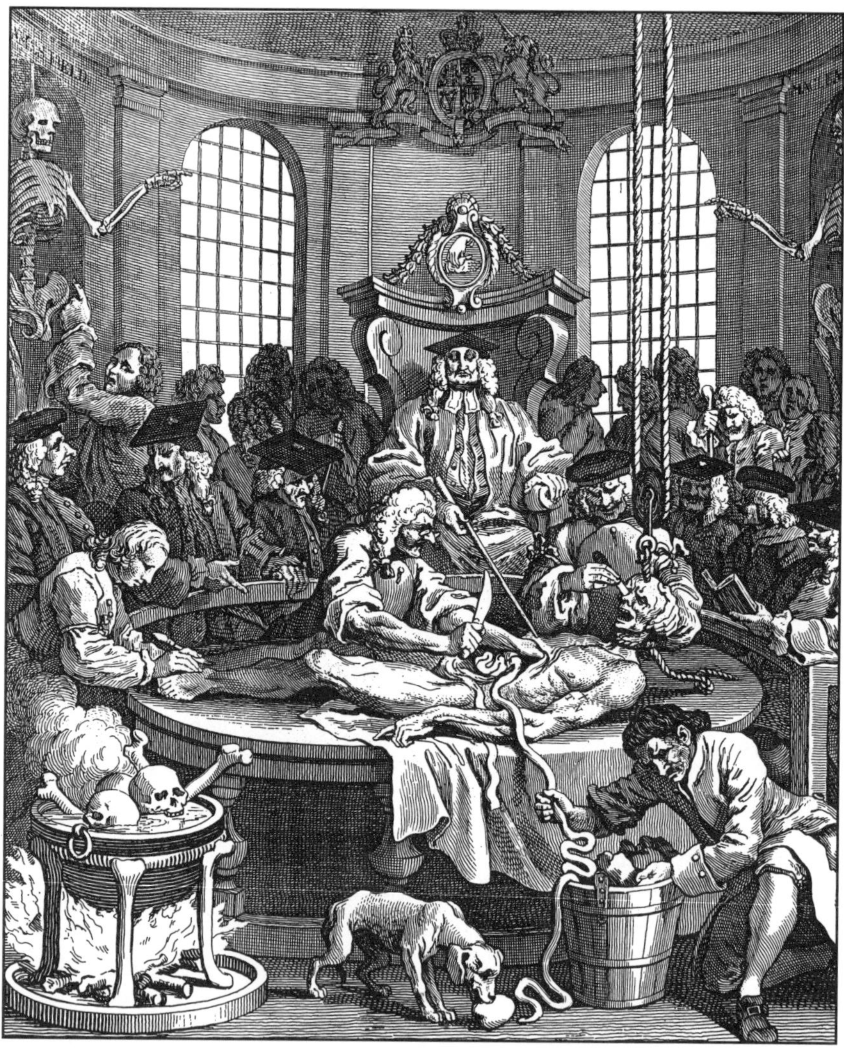

William Hogarth (1697–1764). *The Reward of Cruelty.* Reprinted by permission of Dover Publications, Inc.

Figure 32. **An Eighteenth-Century Autopsy.** In the eighteenth century, progress in anatomical investigation furthered knowledge about the human body. Both pathological changes and underlying structural anomalies were now made visible. These discoveries were shared in an exuberant manner: Autopsies were both legal and public. Anyone could attend the lectures, much as one might attend a concert or a circus in modern times. Criminals were the main source of bodies. In fact, the Murder Act of 1752 in England was established to make punishment appear more horrendous than death alone. In addition to being denied burial, criminals were now publicly dissected after death, and many times criminals were shown the dissected bodies of others prior to their execution. Since most of the people executed were male, science was limited in the number of uteruses it studied.

---

dissections served as family entertainment, much like guillotine beheadings did in France or watching HBO's *Autopsy* series does in the United States (Figure 32). The goal of medical study in Leiden was to "let [students] learne (but not by books but per autopsum) the anatomy of man. . . ."[8]

Universities for teaching medicine sprang up all over Europe. New ways of thinking employed mathematics to prove and test ideas; chemistry and physics were added to the curriculum of European medical schools. Bloodletting was still a part of medical treatment, but eventually Western culture let go of its love affair with barber-surgeon techniques. And important new studies in anatomy appeared in the years of the Enlightenment. In 1762, Giovanni Battista Morgagni wrote *De Sedibus et Causis Morborum per Anatomen Indagatis* (*On the Seats and Causes of Diseases as Investigated by Anatomy*). Morgagni knew his patients well and observed the processes of disease in the living. He later met them one last time on the autopsy table, correlating changes in tissues with the symptoms and signs he remembered. Among the nonscientific community, one of his more appreciated contributions was to discourage the use of frog, toad, and lizard excrement for curative purposes.

Ludmilla Jordanova believes that honesty in representation was an essential element of this period. In her article "Medicine and the Genres of Display," she documents how artists,

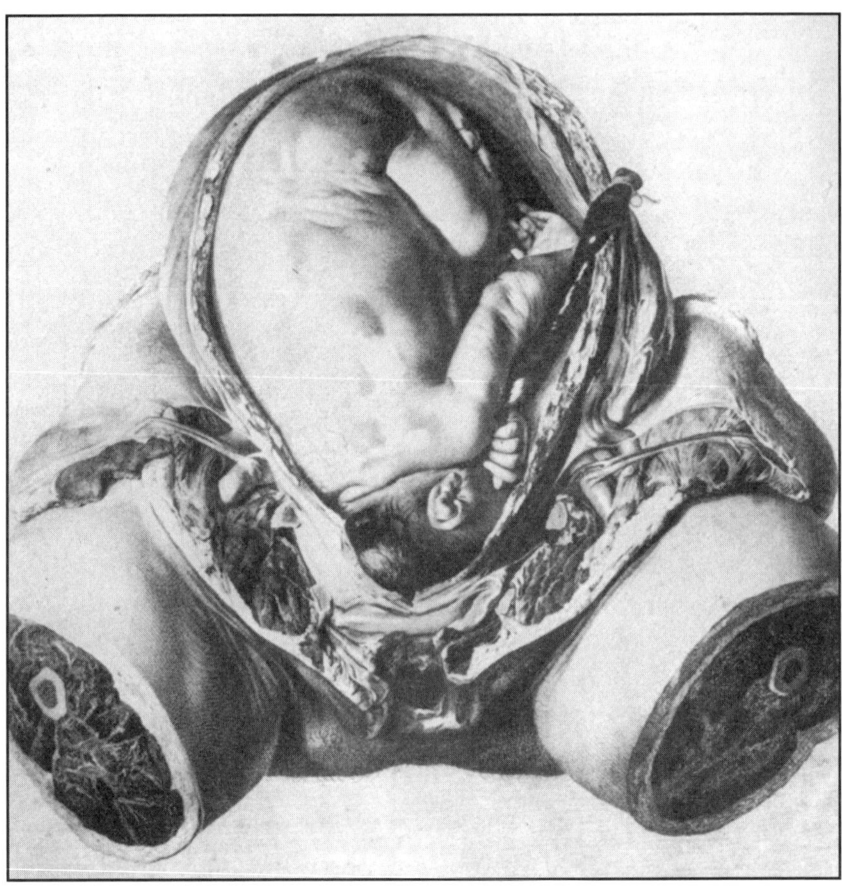

From: Herbert Thoms, M.D., *Classical Contributions to Obstetrics and Gynecology,* 1935. Courtesy of Charles C. Thomas, Publisher, Ltd., Springfield, Illinois.

***Figure 33.* The Eighteenth-Century Uterus.** In 1751, William Hunter, a Scottish surgeon, had the opportunity to prepare the tissues of a third-trimester gravid uterus. As Hunter himself was to note, the gravid uterus was a rarity for anatomists of the time: "One part however, and that the most curious, and certainly not the least important of all, the pregnant womb, had not been treated by [us] with proportionable success" (quoted by Herbert Thoms in *Classical Contributions to Obstetrics and Gynecology*). Hunter made a careful study of the organ and even commissioned ten engraved drawings, each of them meticulously prepared, to accompany his treatise. The preparation was generously made available for the public to view, with much the same attitude as one would today display a new computer to a modern audience.

engravers, and printers all played essential parts in bringing new medical knowledge to the public unaltered by dogma. In 1774, for example, William Hunter published his *Anatomy of the Gravid Uterus* (Figure 33). The specimens Hunter prepared were an important means by which he shared his findings with the public, "making visible [his] concern for the health of less fortunate members of society."[9] (Hunter's uteruses are still on display at the College of Physicians and Surgeons in London.)

The question of male versus female seed (*ovum*) became the subject of an intense debate at this time. Antony van Leeuwenhoek, an early microscopist, wrote that he could see tiny men inside sperm, which he referred to as "animalcules." His theory, called "spermist" and based on the idea of *preformationism,* held that sperm contained the entire new individual, only in miniature. Using microscopy against Leeuwenhoek, Karl von Baer—an anthropologist best known for measuring skulls—argued instead for *epigenesis,* which held that "every animal which springs from the coition of male and female is developed from an ovum and none from a simple formative liquid" (though in "formative liquid," von Baer was referring to menstrual blood).[10] Meanwhile, in Italy, Lazzaro Spallanzani finally proved that spontaneous generation, a theory which held that life could arise from nonlife, was not possible. Armed with the new science, Spallanzani artificially impregnated a dog's uterus, proving that canine sperm was necessary for the event of pregnancy to occur.

A subsequent rise in population accompanied these incredible scientific revelations. Certain reformers viewed this population expansion as potentially harmful, especially in crowded cities where people were involuntarily forced to live and work together. In 1798, Thomas Robert Malthus published his *Essay on the Principle of Population* advocating sexual self-restraint or birth control,[11] though other authors maintain that Malthus only advocated postponing the age of marriage, and that it wasn't until the nineteenth century that Jeremy Bentham promoted contraception with sponges as superior to coitus interruptus.[12]

Others had their own ideas for social improvement. Johann Peter Frank created the first branch of social medicine, which he described in a six-volume work entitled *System einer Vollstandigen Medicinischen Polizey* (*System of Complete Medical Police*), published in 1777.[13] Frank felt that the state should combine its police powers with the power of the physician and work synergistically as two branches of the same system. The first branch, "forensic medicine," would set social-health policy for the citizenry, while the second branch, "medical police," would do the enforcing. Frank's goals included the overburdening of each European uterus to produce its maximum capacity of children because, to ideologues like Frank, an ever-increasing population was looked upon as an asset, even a weapon. Albert Lyons and R. Joseph Petrucelli write that "no detail was too small to escape Frank's attention if it might conceivably affect the future fertility of the state's subjects. Medical police would be authorized to supervise parties, outlaw unhealthy dances like the waltz, enforce periods of rest, and forbid young women to wear corsets and other fashionable articles of clothing that endangered future pregnancies"[14] (Figure 34). In short, women were again to be treated as brood bitches, possessions whose intrinsic value was reproductive. Frank's emphasis on the breeding function of the human female as a class differed dramatically from his proclaimed purpose of keeping whole classes of people out of permanent misery.

Frank's philosophy is an excellent example of both how Enlightenment ideals were applied to social phenomena and how the potential good from such "progress" did not benefit women. In an age that proclaimed the value of reason, the possession of rationality did not extend to women. Lord Chesterfield elucidated this very point in his letters to his son:

> Women , then, are only children of a larger growth; they have an entertaining tattle, and sometimes wit; but for solid reasoning, good sense, I never knew in my life one that had it, or who reasoned or acted consequentially for four and twenty

> hours together. . . . A man of sense. . . . neither consults them about, nor trusts them with serious matters; though he often makes them believe that he does both; which is the thing in the world that they are most proud of. . . . they have in truth but two passions, vanity and love: these are their universal characteristics.[15]

One might hope that Frank's medical police would have had an internal-affairs department to ensure that institutions dedicated to the public health were doing a worthwhile service to the uterus. But a new problem soon developed in these very institutions—iatrogenic disease—and the ability of the medical profession to police itself was minimal at best.

Technology as practiced by midwives had been restricted to crochets (hooks) and extractors used to remove stillborns from the birth canal. Midwives were patient professionals and knew from experience that contractions and babies had their own schedule. Yet there were always a certain percentage of women who died in childbirth, as well as neonates who underwent embryotomies.[16] This, by its very mutilating nature, killed the wedged baby. Forceps were introduced ideologically as a safer, easier-to-handle technology, a way to avoid embryotomies. Later, in the nineteenth century, hospitals became the preferred place for the upper classes, those who could afford to pay. In London, S. W. Fores (who was not a doctor), valiantly pioneered to train intelligent women to be midwives: "He proposed the opening of a school in London where young women might study anatomy, physiology, version and the diseases of women and children. Necessary clinical experience would be obtained through supervised attendance at the deliveries of the poor."[17] But Fores's effort failed, as did other attempts to broaden the social roles of women. Throughout the eighteenth century, as society gained in its ability to understand the world and control it, women were not allowed to take part in this

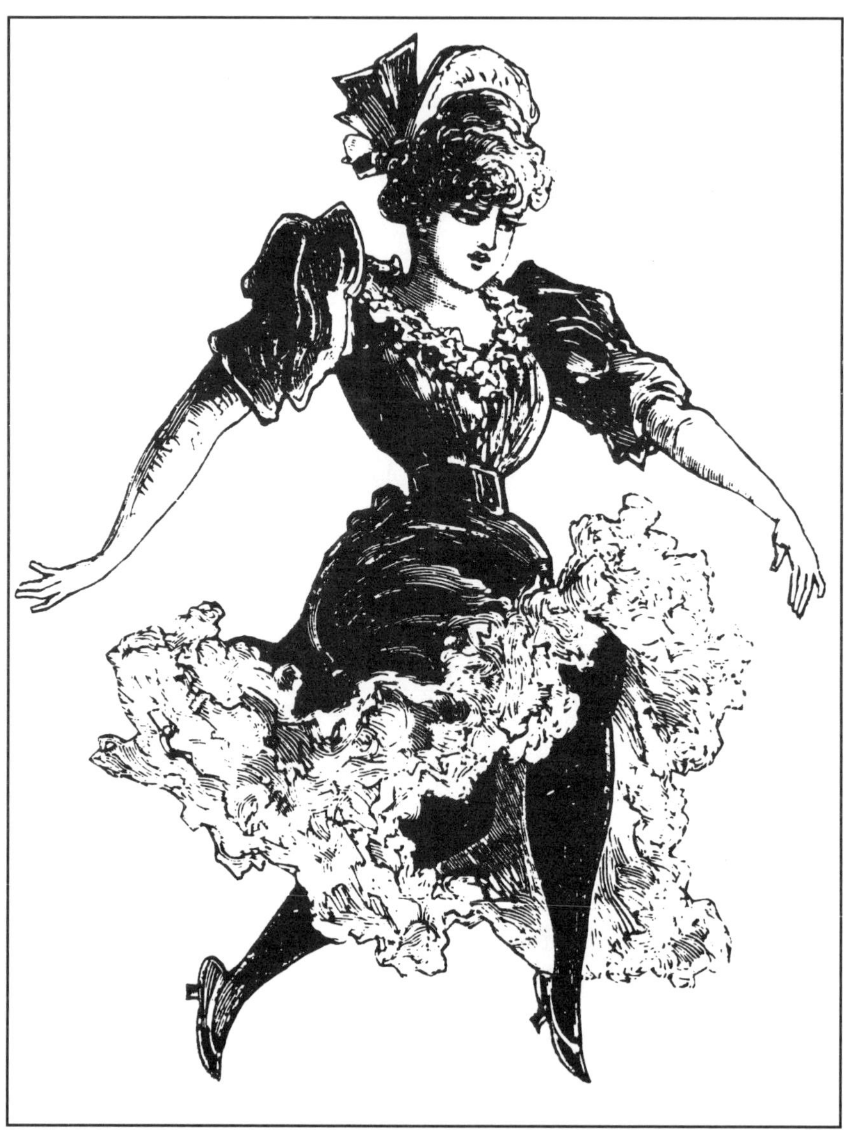

***Figure 34.* Corsets and Women's Bodies.** In 1536, Vesalius examined the body of "an eighteen-year-old girl of noble birth" who was thought to have died from "strangulation of the uterus," and observed that her uterus was normal. He set down his observations as follows:

> From constriction of the thorax, by a corset the girl had been accustomed to wear so that her waist might appear long and willowy, I judged that the complaint lay in a compression of the torso around the hypochondria and lungs. Although she had suffered from an ailment of the lungs, yet the astonishing compression of the organs in the hypochondria appeared to us to be the cause of her ailment, even though we found nothing that would indicate strangulation of the uterus. . . . After the attendant women had left to shed their corsets as quickly as possible . . . I dissected the girl's uterus. . . .

Vesalius concluded that the corset had restricted the girl's breathing so severely that her lungs were unable to expand and aerate normally, and that she had died from pleurisy or some infection in her chest.

Similarly, Johann Peter Frank (1745–1821) wanted to outlaw the corset because he considered it detrimental to the childbearing propensity of the uterus. Yet, each generation and every society has its idealized model of how a woman should look. Since humans express so much genetic variability in physical form, there is an infinite number available. However, a cultural characteristic of humans is that they like to modify those forms with some decoration or mark which identifies them with their culture. During the eighteenth and nineteenth centuries, exaggerated dorsal and lumbar curves in women were preferred. Corsets accentuated these by compressing the midtorso. Unfortunately, by doing so, movement of the breathing apparatus as well as ability to bend and twist were severely compromised. By hyperfeminizing the body, women could be kept in their place figuratively as well as literally.

---

exploration. Education for women was acceptable only if it made them better wives and mothers and more agreeable to men.[18] How strange for this to occur in a time when Rousseau himself had concluded "that if the mind of man at birth is mere receptivity, education can mold intelligence and character with little regard to hereditary differences of mental capacity."[19]

In 1817, when Princess Charlotte Augusta of England died in childbirth at the age of twenty-one—after nearly fifty hours in labor and attended by a male midwife (Figure 35)—the postmortem diagnosis of a "congenital problem" disguised the real

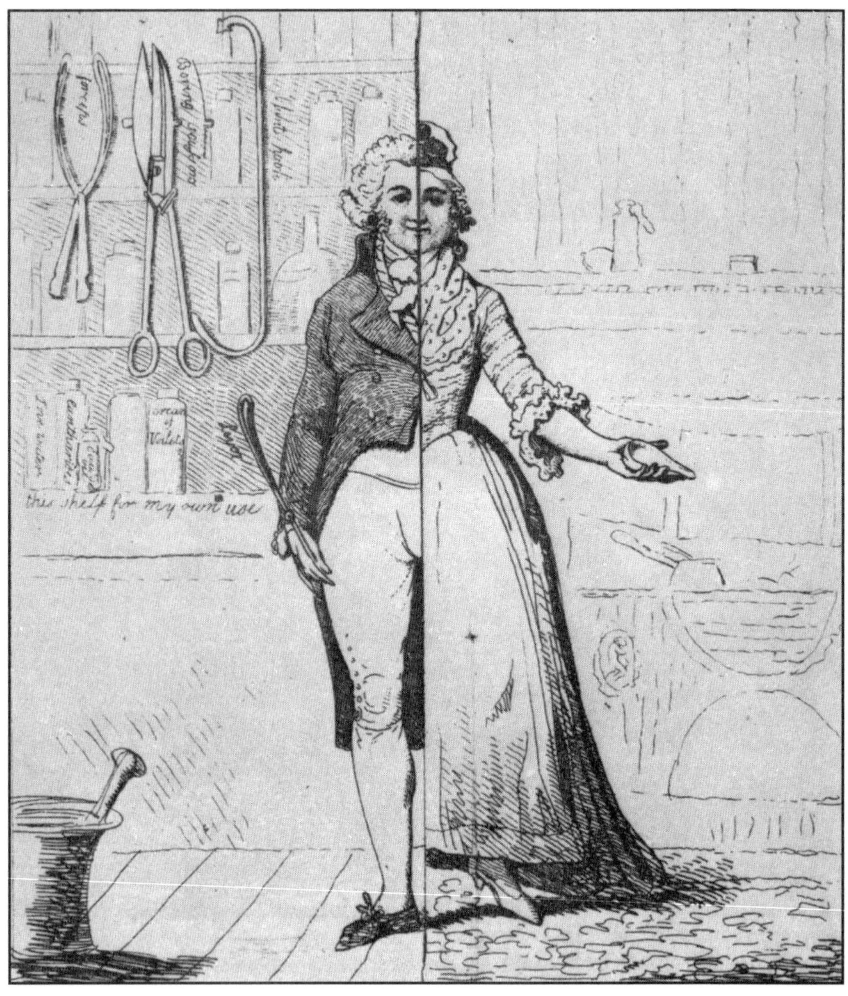

Picture courtesy of Yale University, Harvey Cushing/John Hay Whitney Medical Library.

***Figure 35.* The Male Midwife.** Male midwives were met with ridicule, contempt, and cooperation. The first to employ forceps, they were desired by upper-class women. One belief, as Jane Donegan writes in *Women and Men Midwives,* was that female midwives needed "superior assistance" when they were not physically able to turn a child in utero. Allegedly, women could not cope with crises such as abnormal births or presentations. The surgeon John Maubray, who taught midwifery to his students, is quoted as saying that men "had better presence of mind, were better acquainted with physical helps and could always devise something newer, or give quicker relief in difficult cases than the *common midwife*" (italics mine).

What is strangely referred to in the twentieth century as the "partial-birth abortion" was performed by male midwives. In the eighteenth century, the procedure was known as *embryotomy* and it was performed to save the life of the mother when the baby was wedged in the pelvis, either alive or dead. The male midwife or surgeon would insert his hand into the vagina, find any suture of the infant's skull, place two fingers against it and, using his scissors, enlarge the space, collapsing the skull size so that he could pull the baby out using his fingers as a hook.

Male midwives sometimes were disguised as women so that the woman in labor would not be upset at the thought of a strange man in her birth chamber. Hence, the skirt on the male midwife shown here is both metaphorical and actual.

---

cause of her demise. It is obvious to the modern reader that her medical care, while typical for the time, presented grave risks to her health. The male midwife, Sir Richard Croft, felt the expectant mother should lose some weight. He purged and bled her until she was quite weakened, and when Charlotte did not go into labor on schedule, Croft bled her again. Although the princess desperately wanted to have her mother and a friend present during the delivery, politics did not allow it. Instead, she was attended by the male midwife Croft, as well as the Royal Physician, Dr. Matthew Baillie, and Dr. John Sims, who promised to use forceps if necessary. But after allowing the princess to labor for more than 48 hours without intervention, the doctors delivered a dead heir.[20]

Several hours later, Charlotte was seized with violent abdominal cramps (as well as a ringing in her ears) and died shortly thereafter. In the days that followed, the press was supportive of Croft, Baillie, and Sims, defended their efforts, and attributed the princess's death to a congenital physical problem characterized by "spasms of a violent nature" and the underlying tendency to become excitable under stress (much like the mad king, George III). The autopsy on Charlotte revealed nothing conclusive; but some critics feel that, in this instance, forceps in the hands of experienced midwives probably would have saved the lives of mother and child.[21]

Up until this time, toxicity of the uterus was blamed on something inherently inferior, abnormal, and faulty in women. The natural state of woman, with her menstrual discharges and spoiled seed, had always been synonymous with poison, abnormality, and inferiority. Now an actual putrefaction did exist. But it was not the fault of the uterus; rather, it was the result of doctors who dipped their fingers into cadavers but did not wash their hands before examining women. As more and more women saw hospitals as the safest place to give birth, more and more women died in childbirth as the result of iatrogenic infection.

Gordon of Aberdeen (1752–1799) and Charles White of Manchester (1728–1813), both obstetricians, cautioned midwives and physicians about the contagious nature of puerperal fever. Later, Ignaz Semmelweiss discovered that the cause was carried to patients by doctors, students, or whoever else worked on cadavers, spread from the autopsy room to the delivery room on ungloved fingers and hands. At the Allgemeines Krankenhaus where Semmelweiss worked, women either delivered in the students' ward or the wards attended by midwives. Although the students' ward was more prestigious, the death rate was higher. Semmelweiss published his research, the result of fifteen years of documentation with data taken from three hospitals, which showed that puerperal fever first, was introduced to the uterus or puerpera by decomposing organic animal material; second, was produced by infection from the outside, not by self-infection; and third, was preventable by handwashing. This would have been good news if the importance of asepsis (sterilization) was accepted, but this was not yet a scientific paradigm. Koch and Pasteur had yet to demonstrate that organisms too small to see were responsible for wound infections.[22] Thus the tissues and blood of women with puerperal fever festered, putrefied, and spread to the healthy. The notion that one could prevent such infection simply by washing one's hands seemed absurd. In other words, the uterus was at risk because reason refused to trust a simple pragmatic act. It would take more advanced tools of science to reveal the stuff of which iatrogenic disease was made.

ENDNOTES

1. Richard M. Brace, *The Making of the Modern World* (New York: Holt, Rinehart, 1960), p. 347.

2. Michèle Crampe-Casnabet, "A Sampling of Eighteenth-Century Philosophy." In *A History of Women in the West, Volume 3: Renaissance and Enlightenment Paradoxes,* Georges Duby and Michelle Perrot, eds. (Cambridge: Belknap Press, 1993), p. 326.

3. Natalie Zemon Davis and Arlette Farge, "What Are Women Anyway?" *A History of Women in the West, Volume 3: Renaissance and Enlightenment Paradoxes,* Georges Duby and Michelle Perrot, eds. (Cambridge: Belknap Press, 1993), p. 258.

4. Quoted in Crampe-Casnabet, p. 328.

5. Quoted in R. L. Archer, ed., *Jean-Jacques Rousseau: His Educational Theories, Selected from* Émile, Julie, *and Other Writings* (Woodbury, Conn.: Barron's Educational Series, Inc., 1964), p. 218.

6. Quoted in ibid., pp. 253–54.

7. Quoted in Logan Clendening, ed., *Source Book of Medical History* (New York: Dover Publications, Inc., 1960), p. 281.

8. Harmen Beukers, "Leiden's Medical Faculty During Its First Two Centuries." In *The Anatomy Lesson: Art and Medicine,* Brian T. Kennedy and Davis Coakley, eds. (Dublin: The National Gallery of Ireland, 1992), p. 133.

9. Ludmilla Jordanova, "Medicine and Genres of Display." In *Visual Display: Culture Beyond Appearances,* Lynne Cooke and Peter Wollen, eds. (Seattle: Bay Press, 1995), p. 207.

10. *Dictionary of Scientific Biography, Volume One,* Charles Coulson Gillespie, ed. (New York: Charles Scribner's Sons, 1940), p. 386.

11. David Crystal, "Thomas Robert Malthus." In *The Cambridge Bio-*

graphical Encyclopedia (Cambridge: Cambridge University Press, 1995), p. 614.

12. For a more complete history of condoms, contraception, and birth control, see Vern L. Bullough and Bonnie Bullough, *Sexual Attitudes: Myths and Realities* (Amherst, N.Y.: Prometheus Books, 1995).

13. Albert Lyons and R. Joseph Petrucelli, *Medicine: An Illustrated History* (New York: Harry N. Abrams, Inc., 1987), p. 497.

14. Ibid., p. 497.

15. Quoted in Gordon Allport, *The Nature of Prejudice* (Garden City: Doubleday, 1948), p. 32.

16. *Embryotomy* is a euphemism for the puncture of the fetal fontanelle in order to collapse the skull. This allows a head too large to pass through the pelvic bones to be dislodged. It results in the death of the neonate.

17. S. W. Fores, "Man Midwifery Dissected." Quoted in Jane B. Donegan, *Women and Men Midwives* (Westport, Conn.: Greenwood Press, 1978), p. 172.

18. Martine Sonnet, "A Daughter to Educate." In *A History of Women in the West, Volume 3: Renaissance and Enlightenment Paradoxes,* Georges Duby and Michelle Perrot, eds. (Cambridge: Belknap Press, 1993), p. 110.

19. Will and Ariel Durant, *The Story of Western Civilization, Volume 9: The Age of Voltaire* (New York: Simon and Schuster, 1965), p. 583.

20. Thea Holme, *Prinny's Daughter* (London: Hamish Hamilton, 1976), pp. 235–40.

21. Jane B. Donegan, *Women and Men Midwives* (Westport: Greenwood Press, 1978), pp. 175–76.

22. Clendening, p. 604.

Chapter 7

The Victorian Uterus

When midwifery no longer was helpful to the uterus, "maleness became a necessary attribute of safety, and femaleness became a condition in need of male medical control."[1] But how could a male doctor provide safety if he lacked both personal and professional experience? His reputation was on the line with regard to decision making, yet he had no role model to follow. Under his aegis, childbirth became an initiation rite for himself as well as mother and child. His new role defined normality for parturient women, despite his abnormal way of performing a gynecological examination (Figure 36).

Not everyone trusted medical men doing gynecology and obstetrics (Figure 37). A standard treatment for amenorrhea (the abnormal cessation of menstrual function) was to place leeches directly on the cervix. One might think that a university education would preclude the perpetuation of this bloody practice, but in this case doctors emulated midwives. The bleeding these hungry annelids promoted may have been psychologically sat-

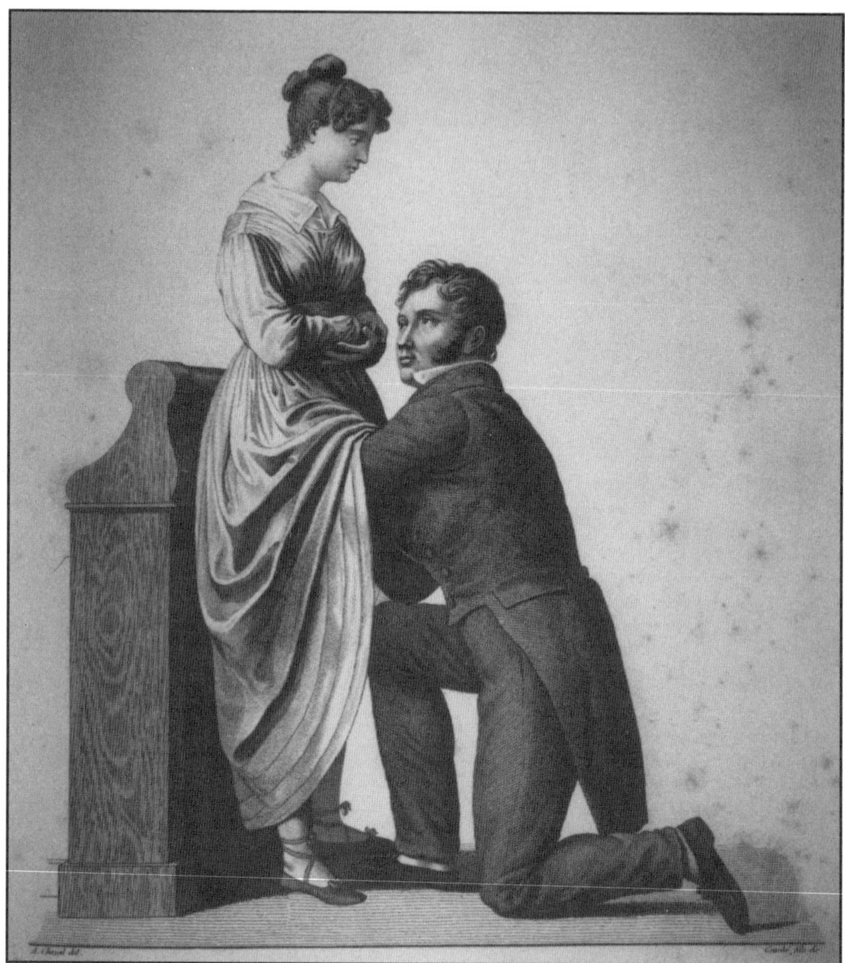

Figure 36. **The Respectable Gynecological Examination.** After men took over the function of midwifery, it became incumbent upon them to learn how to examine a woman's uterus. Mores of the time made this way of examination not only acceptable but required. As Jane B. Donegan notes in her book *Women and Men Midwives,* physicians were instructed not to make eye contact with women but to give them "the idea of making provision for whatever may happen in our absence. We may pass our finger up the vagina or opening to the womb, and make a moderate degree of pressure, for just a few seconds on any part of it, so that she may just feel it; after which we may say to her, 'There ma'am, I have done something that will be of great use to your labor.' "

isfactory, but what happened to the patient the following month? Occasionally a leech would slither into the uterus through the cervical os, with disastrous consequences for the woman. Despite its hazards, bloodletting was still validated as a therapy to rid the body of noxious waste. The pale complexions valued by Victorians could have been the result of the repeated depletion of red blood cells. (Victorian women also made a conscious effort to avoid sunlight or the exertion that might put a blush on the cheeks.) The cult of pure womanhood demanded a frail, indoor woman, weighted down by petticoats and layered yards of ornate fabric.

One prominent Victorian physician who promoted such beliefs was Dr. Frederick Hollick, author of *The Origin of Life and Process of Reproduction in Plants and Animals.* In a chapter entitled "Derangement of the Functions of the Female Organs," Hollick wrote of *chlorosis* or "green sickness":

> The supposed causes of chlorosis are . . . precocious puberty, growing too fast, a feeble constitution, menstrual derangement, melancholy, and mental excitement, and especially certain vicious habits [i.e., masturbation]. The subjects of chlorosis are the most interesting perhaps of all that come under the physician's care. Delicate and sensitive, stricken by a disease from which they deeply suffer, but which often leaves their beauty untouched, or even heightens its attractions, they excite the liveliest emotions of pity, and the most ardent desire to render them assistance.[2]

He goes on to describe hysteria in the next section:

> Almost every woman has either experienced or seen what is called hysterics. . . . Probably the more frequent predisposing causes are, weak constitution, indolence, a city life, bad physical and moral education, the over-excitement of certain feelings . . . it is also most common between puberty and the change of life, but is nevertheless found in quite young girls and in old women . . . those who have deranged menstrua-

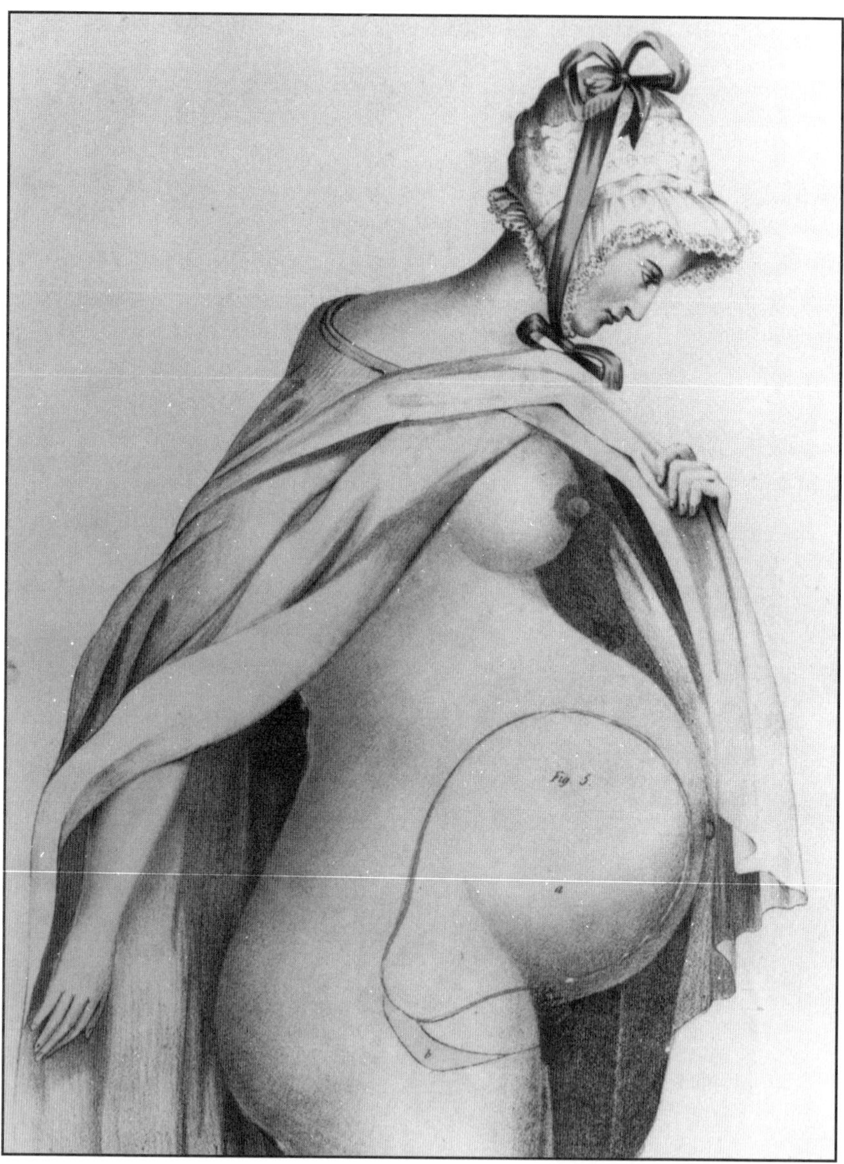

Photo courtesy of Historical Collections, Health Sciences Library, SUNY Health Science Center, Syracuse.

***Figure 37.* The Nineteenth-Century Uterus: Clinical Instruction.** In 1850, a medical doctor who allowed students to watch a childbirth was taken to court for it. The students were accused of salacious stares and meretricious curiosity. The medical profession suffered discord within its ranks over the incident and many publications responded to the event. As Jane B. Donegan reports in her book *Women and Men Midwives,* "The *New York Medical Gazette* agreed that exposure of the patient was never necessary and . . . vaginal exploration, manipulations, delivery by the forceps and embryotomy can all be performed by a competent man without the eye. . . . The Committee on Medical Education felt that there was no need for medical students to use live subjects or to watch a childbirth because there were drawings [such as the one show here]. . . . Demonstrative midwifery was unnecessary." The important thing was that the delivery be in a dignified manner.

> tion, also widows, those who have no children and those in whom the change of life is about to take place. Some of the immediate causes are, the first period, suppressed menstruation, late marriage, chronic inflammation of the womb, vicious habits, and long continued constipation.[3]

The moral remained imbedded in diagnostic categories; as Vern Bullough observes, "a new age of science had given its imprimatur to explanations which tended to reconfirm old religious truths."[4]

Cathartic, purgative, and emetic patent medicines unnecessarily challenged many a woman's healthy alimentary tract while promising to make her a healthier individual. There was a need for milder, less harmful medicine. Enter Lydia E. Pinkham and her Vegetable Compound (Figure 38), advertised as:

> a sure cure for Prolapsus Uteri or falling of the Womb, and all FEMALE WEAKNESSES, including Leucorrhea, Painful Menstruation, Inflammation, and Ulceration of the Womb, Irregularities, Floodings, etc. Pleasant to the taste, efficacious and immediate in its effect, It is a great help in pregnancy, and relieves pain during labor.[5]

It should be pointed out that there is such a condition as a prolapsed uterus, but it results from the ligaments of the uterus

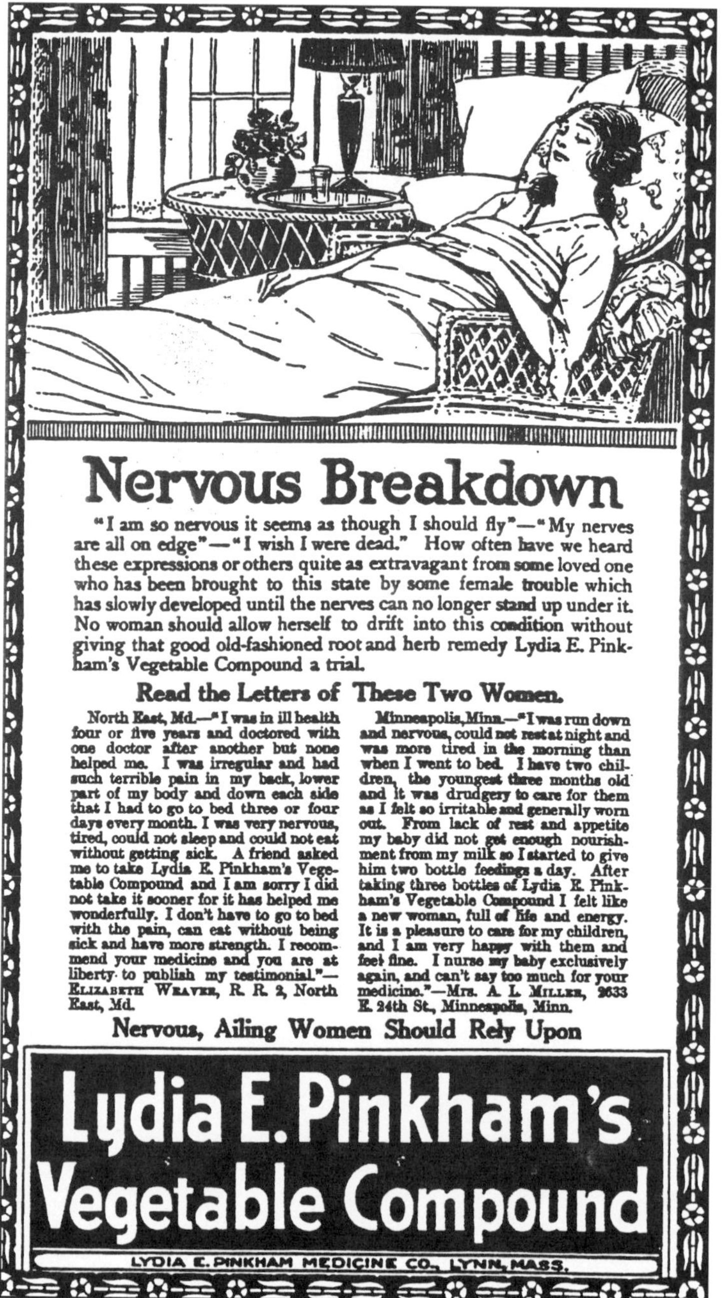

***Figure 38.* Advertisement for Lydia E. Pinkham's Vegetable Compound.**
Courtesy of Schlesinger Library, Radcliffe College.

weakening after repeated pregnancies, trauma during childbirth, or poor postpartum management "which [leaves] the damaged perineum unsewn and weakened."[6] This real problem was quite different from the vague, diffuse plethora of illnesses blamed on a faulty uterus. Undifferentiated uterine problems were also treated by restricting women's choices, whether in apparel, such as lacing, corsets, or fancy dress, or in healthy activities, such as singing, dancing, skating, or horseback riding—not to mention "self-abuse."[7] Nonetheless, Lydia's line of products appealed to the woman who aspired to the "cult of pure womanhood" and was perhaps abnormal, unfulfilled, or pregnant. The subsequent promoter of Pinkham's products was a man who wrote under the name "Dorothy Grey" and made such wise statements as "Trouble lies in our physical rather than our social condition," "Every woman who feels dissatisfied with her lot should realize that she is sick and should take steps to make herself well," and "Mrs. Pinkham's medicine will make a woman more ready to meet the wishes of her husband." He also promised that by dosing herself with Mrs. Pinkham's, a woman would be enabled to find "her true vocation—to be a devoted wife and loving mother."

Although the Lydia E. Pinkham marketing campaign and product line may seem terribly unsophisticated, it was an attempt to bring self-care to a population of women who wanted control of their own bodies. Lydia E. Pinkham's Sanative Wash, for example, was introduced ostensibly as a hygienic douche, but really was meant to be used as a form of birth control. Why the guise? To elude the vigilance of Anthony Comstock, a self-appointed moral guardian of the day who was obsessed with such "traps of Satan" as alcohol, gambling, prostitution, and obscenity. Contraceptives and abortifacients were in the same category as pornography in his epistemology. Like Augustine, Comstock considered nonprocreative sexuality "bestial and base."[8] He was able to pressure the 1873 session of Congress into voting to criminalize any written material dealing with pornography, contraception, abortifacients, or free love.[9] So formidable was his political clout that only two senators and one congressman dared to question the way the measure was passed. (By a voice vote.)

Why did this ludicrous law become reality? Politically, Comstock was in the right place for an ultraconservative after the Civil War. Validated by the YMCA, he devoted himself originally to "saving America's youth from the devil's temptations."[10] His code lumped materials deemed obscene, lewd, lascivious, indecent, immoral, and filthy together with contraception, abortion, and information about sex—a mixed bag, but nonetheless an agenda that few would dispute. Coupled with a social atmosphere in which childbearing was allegedly the ultimate fulfillment of every woman, the Comstock laws attempted to foil the potential evil of "free love" and to reinforce the values of self-restraint and woman's subordinate place. In the nineteenth century, a "true woman" did not step outside of her proper sphere (home, family, and children). Women were born to become mothers, and those who did not were blighted, physically as well as emotionally.[11]

That same year (1873), Edward H. Clarke warned that if women were admitted to Harvard, it would be detrimental to their health: Education, he argued, would cause their wombs to atrophy.[12] In Clarke's view, although women had the right to do what they were capable of doing, "one of the things they could not do and still retain their good health was to be educated on the pattern and model of men."[13] Womb power was inversely related to brain power, and those who suggested otherwise paid the price. Once such person was Edward Bliss Foote, "the proponent of womb veils [a form of contraception] and a popular health writer," who, as Ellen Chesler records, "was convicted by Comstock and forced to reissue his advice book on contraception in a truncated version that only advertised douching" instead of more instructive information.[14]

The French historian Michelet characterized the nineteenth century as the Age of the Womb, but readers of this book know better. Every century has been the Age of the Womb as far as the control of women is concerned. From fallen wombs and compressed organs to hysteria, dancing mania, melancholia, love sickness, puerperal fever, and the pathological aura that defines woman, female anatomy has been the cause. (Michelet himself "regarded the womb as a tyrannical organ 'encompassing, within its dominion, almost the entire range of woman's actions and affections.' ")[15] In the nineteenth century, the "healthy functioning of a woman's organs was a measure of her personal and social worth," according to Richard and Barbara Wertz, and the phrase "female complaints" became a generic term used to describe any health problem.[16] (It also had a moral overlay, reflecting some social or personal inadequacy on the part of the woman with the complaint). Thus, Dr. M. E. Dirix could write in 1869 that "headaches to sore throats, curvature of the spine, bad posture, or pains anywhere in the lower half of the body could be the result of 'displacement' of the womb." Dr. Dirix continued:

> Thus women are treated for diseases of the stomach, liver, kidneys, heart, lungs, etc.; yet, in most instances, these diseases will be found, on due investigation, to be, in reality, no diseases at all, but merely the sympathetic reactions or the symptoms of one disease, namely, a disease of the womb.[17]

Upper-class women could use medical excuses to avoid housework or child care. The rest cure of H. Weir Mitchell played into this mutually reinforcing relationship between greedy physicians and women who wished to emotionally blackmail their husbands. Sarah Stage observes that "through illness, an unhappy wife could create some limited identity and demand attention and affection from a husband too often absent."[18] Dr. Mitchell's popular brand of therapy/punishment was scrutinized in Charlotte Perkins Gilman's famous short story "Yellow Wallpaper," in which a woman writer, married to a doctor, is forced to take the rest cure to rid herself of those mental activities and intellectual pursuits that interfere with marriage and motherhood. In a reverse twist, she is cured when she divorces her husband and marries her writing career. But Gilman's heroine was the exception. If women were apt to succumb to illness, they were unfit to be admitted into professions where they could compete with men—and the more status the position held, the more their entry was resisted. As Vern Bullough observes, it was no coincidence that "medical opposition to feminine emancipation began to increase as the physician himself felt threatened by the few women attempting to enter medical school."[19]

In her critical survey of American medicine, Gina Corea records how the medical establishment attempted to rationalize the exclusion of women:

> Male doctors . . . asserted that menstruation, pregnancy, childbirth and menopause were illnesses. Healthy men certainly never experienced them. These functions were such severe disabilities that they, along with woman's general weakness, precluded well-paid work. For their health's sake, women would have to keep out of job competition, marry and remain dependent on men.[20]

With regard to menstruation, Dr. Frederick Hollick opined that "this function alone makes it impossible for women, except in a few peculiar individual cases, to pursue the same mode of life as man. It makes her, of necessity, not so continuously active, nor so capable of physical toil, while at the same time . . . [causes her] to yearn for sympathy and support from some being that she feels is more powerful than herself."[21]

The door to education and economic independence was closed to women, especially those of the middle class and above. Marriage was touted as the future of all females. Women could avoid sex by being "unwell," and since all women were unwell at least once a month, their "inherent illness" and "abnormal physiology" justified industry's refusal to pay them as much as men for equal work.

It should be emphasized, however, that not all employment

was off limits. Unskilled, low-paying, servile jobs such as maid, housekeeper, or servant were open to women, especially women of color. They didn't stress the brain at the expense of the uterus. Interestingly, as garment cottage industries were replaced by factory jobs, rank and prestige mirrored conventional male-female familial relations. Men were in charge and women were subservient, required to ask permission and told how to behave and work.

Since birth control was neither an option nor available, pregnancy after marriage was all but inevitable. Once a woman's uterus was implanted with a zygote, her body was no longer her own. She belonged to society and she was now guardian of a new life. Abortion was off limits as well and the moral horrors of its consequences articulated clearly, as in this "advice" from George H. Napheys:

> WARNING: If maternal sentiment is so callous in their breasts, let them know that such produced abortions are the constant cause of violent and dangerous womb disease, and frequently of early death, that they bring on mental weakness and often insanity. . . . Better, far better to bear a child every year for twenty years, than to resort to such wicked and injurious steps; better to die, if needs be, in the pangs of childbirth, than to live with such a weight of sin on the conscience.[22]

By making motherhood the highest form of female achievement, a tremendous shame was placed on those who did not conceive. As Carroll Smith-Rosenberg and Charles Rosenberg have written, "Motherhood was woman's normal destiny and those females who thwarted the promise immanent in their body's design must expect to suffer."[23] When a married woman did not become pregnant, the details of her bedroom behavior were analyzed ad nauseam. One article about sterility, published in 1891, blamed anything that tended to hasten, prevent, or retard orgasm as the reason for the nonunion of egg and sperm. Perfect orgasm (defined as simultaneous orgasm) was thought to possess the power to impregnate. At the same time, however, since sexual desire was thought to be weaker in the female than in the male, orgasm in women was considered an unnatural phenomenon.

The presumed relationship between impregnation and orgasm had never been empirically tested in the centuries since Renaissance writers had first stated it as fact. Now it presented a moral dilemma, because if orgasm was unnatural in women but was nonetheless necessary for conception (and if the ideal women was to conceive as often as possible), how were women supposed to respond to sexual stimulation?

Another cause for concern was the fact that educated women were choosing to have fewer children and were getting pregnant later in life. According to Dr. Thomas W. Kay, writing in the February 7, 1891, issue of the *Journal of the American Medical Association,* this was "due to the development of the cerebrum at the expense of the cerebellum . . . judging from their crania, the 'organ of phyloprogenitiveness' was poorly developed." In Dr. Kay's view, prostitutes could avoid pregnancy by not allowing orgasm to take place. He also cited the example of a married woman who avoided disease by not "allowing her passions to be aroused," and who avoided pregnancy as well by "bearing down and forcing out the seminal fluid after the act [had] been accomplished."[24]

Another reason for delayed pregnancy in educated women had to do with the peculiar effects of brainwork itself. Vern Bullough and Martha Voght report that according to J. H. Kellogg, "Many young women have permanently injured their constitutions while at school by excessive mental taxation during the catamenial period." Another physician, F. W. Van Dyke,

> claimed that hard study killed sexual desire in women, took away their beauty, and brought on hysteria, neurasthenia, dyspepsia, astygmatism, and dysmenorrhea. Educated women, he added, could not bear children with ease because study

> arrested the development of the pelvis at the same time it increased the size of the child's brain and therefore its head.[25]

These pseudoscientific statements were not challenged too much at first because their proponents were highly respected in other areas of the medical profession.

One might think that if menstruation and pregnancy were indications of illness, then once this pattern ended, women would be considered cured. But no—Colombat d'Isère said that, at menopause, the female "becomes sad, restless, taciturn, she regrets her lost power to please."[26] Women at that stage were advised to retire to a "quiet life" and "withdraw from the world." Like her menstruating sister, the post-menopausal woman was expected to adhere to the "cult of true womanhood."

The "true woman" of the nineteenth century was "delicate, timid, and in need of protection." She was also soft spoken, gentle, and pure, yet "fulfilled the domestic agenda of running a good home and caring for her children."[27] She was expected to be obedient to and please her husband, and to be a good (and prolific) mother: "By producing many children, especially many sons, she was able to influence the developing society. . . . These young men would . . . become a reflection of her good mothering."[28] If a woman could not please her husband, or rebelled in any way other than passive resistance, she was given a medical diagnosis of insanity or neurosis. If she experienced sexual pleasure or demonstrated active eroticism, her abnormality was diagnosed as nymphomania. With this paradigm, psychiatry became a powerful tool for controlling and punishing women.

The horror of eighteenth-century lying-in rooms was equaled by nineteenth-century insane asylums. When women failed to live up to their unrealistic roles, psychiatric diagnosis provided a way for a dissatisfied husband to remove his wife from his home to an institution but still have control over her. There were primary and secondary etiologies of insanity as well as secondary symptoms of primary causes. Dr. E. Jarvis, writing

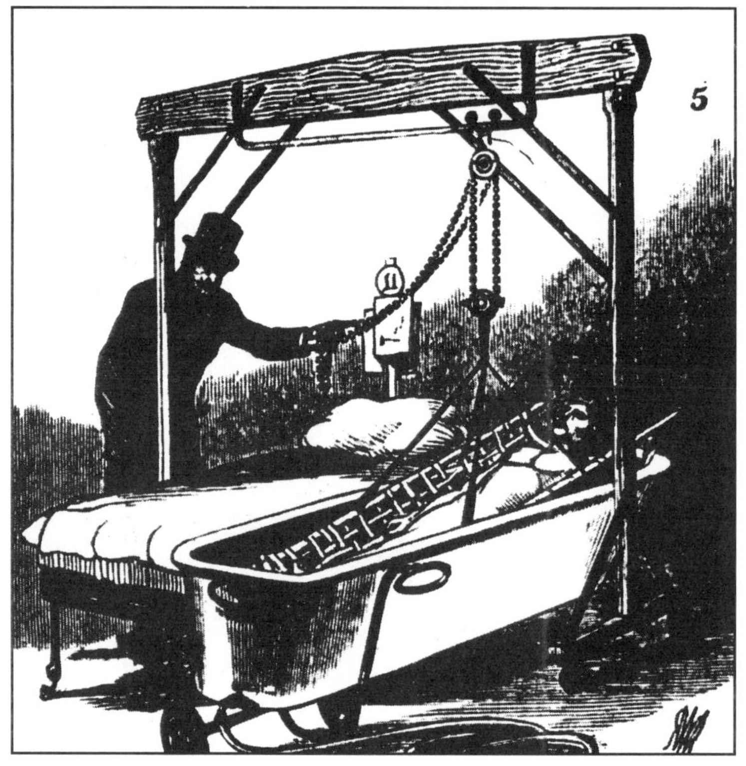

in the *Boston Medical and Surgical Journal* in 1851, listed excessive study, disappointment, and grief as primary causes of female insanity.[29] The gender-specific physical cause of insanity was "a defect in the ovarian or uterine system which produced secondary symptoms of disorganization and hysteria. . . . . Menstruating, giving birth, and lactating were identified as primary causes of secondary insanity in women."[30] In other words, being female was a condition that at any time could be used to augment a psychiatric diagnosis of mental illness. Male doctors echoed Hippocrates when they stated that "marriage remedies and restores debilitated health," and that "pregnancy is a preservative of female health." Insanity in women happened when women "chose to leave the limited sphere of the home,"

***Figure 39.* The Cold-Water Treatment for Hysteria.** Like Bruegel's peasants, who were thrown off the bridge into a cold stream for hysteria, nineteenth-century woman were subjected to the cold-water treatment. If women dared to express a desire to become educated, felt unfulfilled, or verbalized negativity toward domestic responsibilities, they were diagnosed as insane, mad, and conveniently sequestered in asylums. One treatment consisted of stripping a woman of her clothing, immobilizing her with a sheet wrapped around her body, tying her to a cot, and immersing her in a tub of icy water, as shown here.

The use of this type of therapy persisted well into the twentieth century. In their book *Women of the Asylum,* Jeffrey Geller and Maxine Harris offer an account of the ordeal suffered by actress Frances Farmer, as related in her own words: "The orderly unlocked my restraints. 'Prep her for hydro,' she called after us. Before I could organize myself, the trustee had taken down three canvas straps from a hook on the wall and looped one around my chest, pinning my arms against my sides until my breath was cut short. The second was buckled around my thighs and the third around my ankles. She left the room as I tottered to keep my balance. I tried to hop after her but tumbled headlong. My chin cracked against the floor and I felt a sharp pain as my teeth sliced my lower lip. I lay there screaming. . . . They picked me up, one by the ankles, the other by the shoulders, and dropped me into the empty tub, bruising my spine.

"They pulled the heavy canvas sheet up to my neck, and while one tightened the neck drawstring, the other took a long dirty rope and looped it under the lip of the tub. The first crash of icy water hit my ankles and slipped rapidly up my legs. I began to shake from the shock of it, screaming and thrashing my body under the sheet, but the more I struggled, the more I realized that I was helplessly restricted to a frozen hell.

"I began to gnaw on my lip, flinching from the pain of my teeth digging into the wound but praying that it would take my mind off the freezing water that burned my body like acid. . . . Hydro was a violent and crushing method of shock treatment. . . . What it really did was assault the body and horrify the mind until both withered with exhaustion. . . . I lay there in the glacier grip until my mind had gone blank. I felt it slipping from me, but I tried to keep it active by thinking of addresses, phone numbers, nursery rhymes. I counted forward and backward. I became confused. I recited the alphabet, but everything was jumbled. I struggled, and screamed, and froze. Then I slid out of awareness and tumbled into a gibbering, scrambled maze."

"failed to fulfill the roles of wife and mother," or "followed occupations and professions for which they were not suited." In the opinion of nineteenth-century medical researchers, such "unfeminine activities caused uterine derangement which in turn caused mental illness."[31]

In *Women of the Asylum: Voices From Behind the Walls,* authors Jeffrey L. Geller and Maxine Harris profile the case histories of seventeen women who were locked up by their husbands, brothers, fathers, or other male relatives between 1840 and 1945. Once inside those institutions, tortures equivalent to those used in concentration camps were employed to change their behavior. A favorite was the use of cold water, either poured over the head of a patient or used in a tub for soaking; the patient would be confined in a layer of sheets and restrained (Figure 39; the reader is also referred to chapter 1, Figure 3, for an earlier version of this treatment).

Some reasons for involuntary incarceration were ideological. One inmate reported that "my religion was different than my family"; another attributed her problems to "humors in the blood, bad humors"; and still another was locked up because she "could not fall in with every belief that was fashionable." Elizabeth Parsons Ware Packard "defended religious opinions that conflicted with others," and Tirzah F. Shedd was punished for her "monomania or spiritualism." Adriana Brinckle was accused of being "extravagant and too fond of dress." Her family preferred an insanity plea rather than a court trial for an extremely minor, rather ambiguous "offense": She bought furniture on credit and then sold it. Lydia A. Smith, incarcerated from 1865 to 1871 and thus painfully aware of the power differential in marriage, offered this assessment: "If a man tires of his wife and is befooled after some other woman, it is not a very difficult matter to get her in an institution of this kind. Belladonna and chloroform will give her the appearance of being crazy enough."[32]

The uterine-brain connection was documented in other maladies as well. Take the case of "lactational insanity": Dr. Levinstein-Schlegel blamed this disorder on the displacement of the pelvic organs and stated "that local [pelvic] irritations acting upon the central organ [brain] are active, both as determining the duration as well as the course of the mental disorder."[33] The problems of female singers were addressed in another article which read, in part, "when we consider the intimate connection of the uterus with the great sympathetic nervous system, it stands to reason that an inflamed or conjested [*sic*] uterus will, at other times, also prejudiciously affect the organs of voice and song." The author, whose name is not given, emphatically related that he was "positive" of his diagnosis, "for I have time and again witnessed their reflex action on several of my patients. . . . Mrs. S., 40 years of age, suffered from a large uterine fibroid. She had this reflex laryngeal spasm to that extent that suffocation was imminent at each application of anything to the endometrium."[34] The author went on to state that "the immediate and direct connection of the uterine nerves with those of the larynx was conclusively shown, dozens of times, to the students that were with me at my clinics whenever this patient would call."[35]

Like medieval cloistered women, nineteenth-century women were not supposed to speak. If a woman dared to express her thoughts, feelings, or ideas, she was severely reprimanded; to speak publicly was sinful and indicated promiscuous inclinations. When peer pressure and oppression were ineffective, a procedure called glossodectomy could be performed to render her unable to articulate words correctly. This surgical modification cut the tongue in a way that allowed the woman to chew her food and not choke to death, but would render her embarrassed to speak. Like most injustices committed on less powerful social groups, the perpetrators used biblical rhetoric as their justification. Dr. John Scoffern, for example, cited the biblical phrase "If thy right hand offend thee, cut it off" as

> the connection between sinning and the organic cause of sinning; the alliance indicated by Christ. . . . If a tongue res-

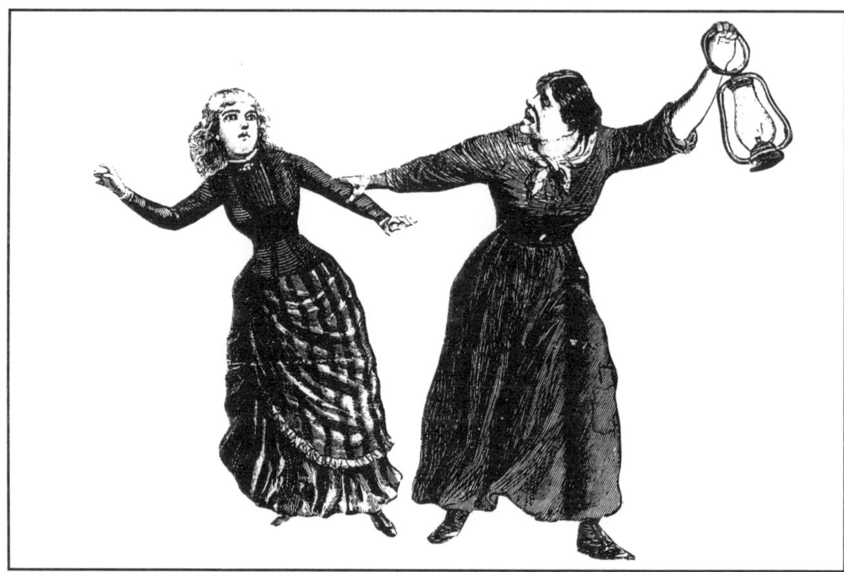

***Figure 40.* Suspicious Signs of the Masturbator.** John Harvey Kellogg, best known today as the inventor of Kellogg's Corn Flakes, ran a popular nineteenth-century sanitarium in Battle Creek, Michigan. Kellogg sought to improve the health of his patients by curbing what he considered unhealthy and excessive sexual desires. What follows is his list of the tell-tale signs of the child masturbator (as quoted in Vern and Bonnie Bullough's *Sexual Attitudes: Myth and Realities*): "General debility; consumption-like symptoms; premature and defective development; sudden changes in disposition; lassitude; sleeplessness; failure of mental capacity, fickleness; untrustworthiness; love of solitude; bashfulness; unnatural boldness; mock piety; being easily frightened; confusion of ideas; aversion to girls in boys but a decided liking for boys in girls; round shoulders; weak backs and stiffness of the joints; paralysis of the lower extremities; unnatural gait; bad position in bed; lack of breast development in females; capricious appetite; fondness for unnatural and hurtful or irritating articles (such as salt, pepper, spice, vinegar, mustard, clay, slate pencils, plaster and chalk); disgust at simple foods; use of tobacco; unnatural paleness; acne or pimples; biting of fingernails; shifty eyes; moist cold hands; palpitation of the heart; hysteria in females; chlorosis or the 'green sickness'; epileptic fits; bed-wetting; and the use of obscene words and phrases." The Bulloughs conclude that in Kellogg's view, "the dangers [of masturbation] were terrible to behold, since genital excitement produced intense congestion and led to urethral irritation, enlarged prostate in males, bladder and kidney infection, priapism, piles and prolapse of the rectum, atrophy of the testes, variococele, nocturnal emissions, and general exhaustion."

> olutely bent on evil speaking be excised, that tongue can speak ill no more. . . . The triumph of psychological surgery is seen in this mild, peripheral, and subcutaneous operation. . . . The patient being under the effects of chloroform, a very fine knife is run though the tongue and rapidly withdrawn. The result is that certain muscular fibres are cut; the mobility of the organ is in some measure impaired,—to the extent, namely, of making continuous and violent objurgation impossible, but not of interfering with any temperate conversation.[36]

Scoffern concluded that the results of the operation force the patient "to conform to the behaviour expected of a woman by making it impossible for her to do anything else."

Glossodectomy was not the ultimate punishment for unnatural female behavior. The book *Surgical Diseases of Women,* written in 1854 by Baker Brown, a student of Guy's Medical College and a founder of St. Mary's in London, documented cases of insanity caused by "self-abuse." According to Dr. Brown, masturbation was an unhealthy practice that caused debility and even insanity; he referred to it as "peripheral excitement" and felt that it was the essence of female insanity.[37] To counteract this dangerous behavior, Dr. Brown perfected the clitoridectomy, a surgical procedure to remove the offending organ. Similarly, Dr. Hollick's book (previously mentioned) included a chapter entitled "The Diseases of Women Familiarly Explained," in which he wrote of the unnatural growth of the clitoris after puberty. Dr. Hollick was convinced that an enlarged clitoris was likely to lead to immorality, and that "attention should be paid immediately to these cases, because they have not only a tendency often to become much worse, but even to degenerate into gangrene, fungus, or cancer." His treatments for this condition included leeches, scarification, or excision; he did allow, however, that "cold water and entire absence from all excitement whatever, is often all that is required."[38] Dr. Marion Sims, famous for doing surgical experimentation on black slaves, amputated the clitoris of a twenty-four-year-old

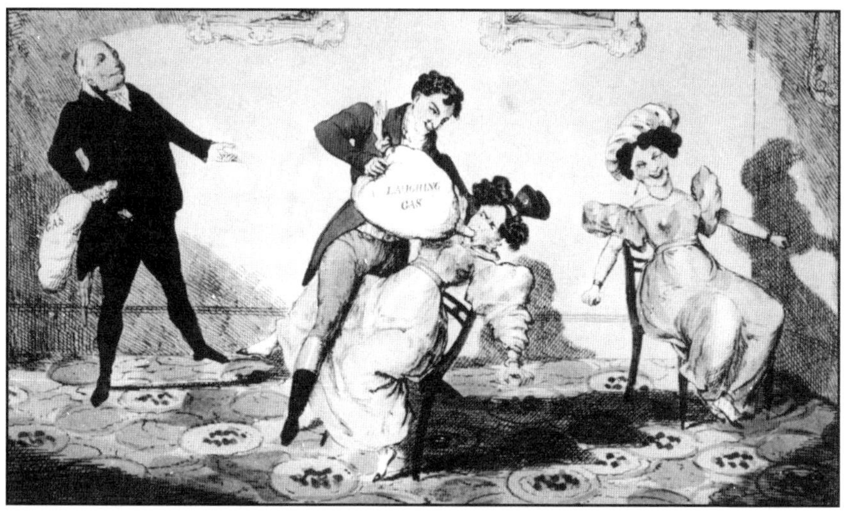

Courtesy of National Library of Medicine, Bethesda.

***Figure 41.* The Original Use of Laughing Gas.** Nitrous oxide was a parlor amusement for men before it was adopted for use in medicine. Here Victorian husbands demonstrate how to make women compliant and passive in a print entitled "Prescription for Scolding Wives." About ten years after the creation of this print, nitrous oxide was used for anesthesia.

woman who was unmarried and had painful periods, convulsions, and bladder irritation for the relief of her nervous or hysterical condition, as recommended by Baker Brown.[39] She afterward was cured of all her problems and never again exhibited symptoms suggestive of uterine dysfunction. Female masturbation was also called "moral leprosy" by A. J. Block, and T. Spratling recommended "nothing short of ovariotomy" for insane females.[40] As can be seen from this brief history, female genital mutilation is not a procedure exclusively practiced by the "other," those pastoral populations north of the equator in Africa. Between about 1850 and 1950, the "age of masturbatory insanity," medical experts advised that self-abuse was dangerous, immoral, unhealthy, and should be eradicated. There was a variety of suspicious signs (Figure 40),[41] and many girls

Courtesy of National Library of Medicine, Bethesda.

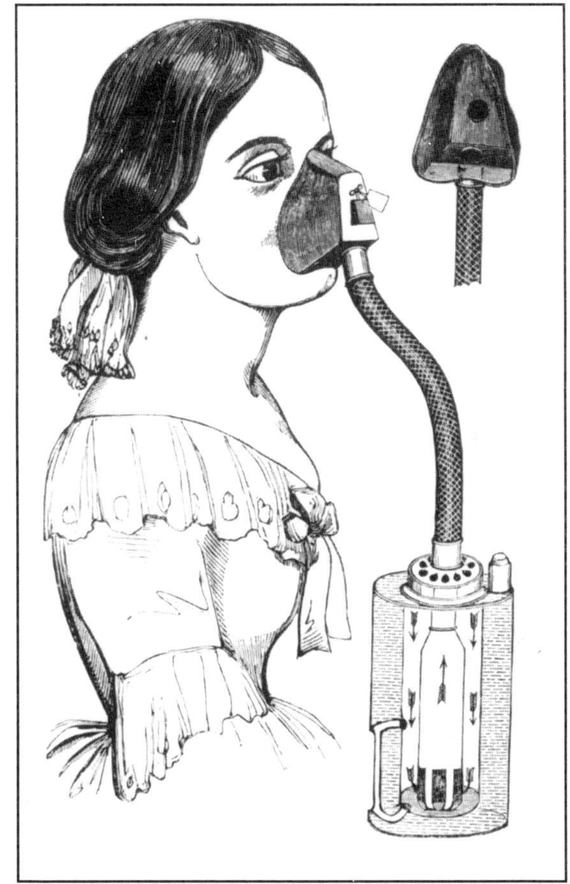

***Figure 42.* Chloroform Mask.** Although anesthetic, in the form of nitrous oxide, was used as a parlor amusement among men who wanted to quiet or change the mood of their wives, its medical use for pain control, particularly in childbirth, was not widespread until after John Snow used it for Queen Victoria. James Young Simpson, a physician who studied in Scotland, published his "Answer to the Religious Objections Advanced against the Employment of Anaesthetic Agents in Midwifery and Surgery" in 1849. He used arguments based on etymological analysis of the words "suffer," "labor," and "pain" in the Bible, as well as arguments that when the rib of Adam had been removed in Genesis, his deep sleep was caused by God, and that other important medical discoveries, such as the smallpox vaccination, had also been deemed diabolical. And if narcosis for pain control in men using oral agents such as opium had already been accepted, Simpson asked, what difference did delivery by the lungs make?

were treated for them with various types of ablation of the clitoris every bit as horrifying as what happens in Africa. Similarly, what we have come to accept as normal with regard to male circumcision is an outgrowth of the fear that a mother handling her infant son's genitalia might stimulate him and induce him to become a chronic masturbator.

The mixing of the moral and the medical is ingrained in health care from cradle to casket. It requires a painstaking dissection of those ideas to separate the two or at least examine why certain attitudes are difficult to dismiss. One of these attitudes involved the use of anesthesia/analgesia in childbirth. When gas was first adopted by the medical profession from show-business chemists, dentists, and peripatetic professors, its use was questioned on philosophical grounds.[42] It was perfectly acceptable to use laughing gas on women if it was administered to control their assertive or independent behavior. (Figure 41) To use it in childbirth was "vehemently condemned by the Calvinist church fathers as contrary to the Biblical admonition that a woman must bring forth her child in pain."[43] Some nineteenth-century medical men maintained that pain was the punishment inflicted by God for people's wickedness, and that anesthesia was "a Satanic plot to deprive men of the capacity to reason and endure the pain that God intended them to experience"[44] (Figure 42). As Lois Magner explains:

> Pain had a God-given and therefore holy role to play in the lives of men, and especially in the lives of women. Midwives had been put to death for the blasphemous, sinful, unnatural crime of attempting to alleviate the pains of childbirth .... Suffering was inherent in female physiology, and labor pains enhanced woman's capacity for tenderness, femininity, and maternal feelings.[45]

Indeed, when Sir James Young Simpson found chloroform to be a better anesthetic than ether and attempted to use it for childbirth, he was met with condemnation from his peers "and assorted moralists." Among the objections Simpson encountered was the assertion that anesthesia lifted the patient's "sexual inhibitions, creating situations in which the lying-in room was . . . defiled by the most painful and obscene conversation and sexual orgasm was substituted for natural pains."[46] Simpson was no fool, however, and promptly found justifications in the Bible for the use of anesthesia. He cited Genesis 3:14–19 and argued,

> If some physicians hold that they feel conscientiously constrained not to relieve the agonies of a woman in childbirth, because it was ordained that she should bring forth [children] in sorrow, then they ought to feel conscientiously constrained on the very same grounds not to use their professional skill and art to prevent man from dying; for at the same time it was decreed . . . that man should be subject to death, "dust thou art, and unto dust shalt thou return."

Simpson also argued that the word "sorrow," in the Hebrew original, could be construed as meaning not "pain" but "muscular effort, toil, or labour":

> The Hebrew word for "labour" [is] used to describe the act of parturition in the lower animals . . . [and] the great characteristic of human parturition is the vastly greater amount of muscular effort, toil, or labour required for its accomplishment. The state of anesthesia does not withdraw or abolish that muscular effort, toil, or labour; for if so, then it would stop, and arrest entirely the act of parturition itself. But it removes the physical pain and agony otherwise attendant on these muscular contractions and efforts.[47]

Simpson also pointed out that many other scientific discoveries were initially opposed on religious grounds, including the vaccination for smallpox, and that the "first surgical operation ever performed on man" was when God removed a rib from Adam after causing a deep sleep to fall on him: "The passage is principally striking as evidence of our Creator himself using means to save poor human nature from the unnecessary endurance of physical pain." It might be said that Simpson paved the way for the subsequent acceptance of obstetrical analgesia with his clever exegesis.

ENDNOTES

1. Richard W. Wertz and Dorothy C. Wertz, *Lying-In: A History of Childbirth in America* (New Haven, Conn.: Yale University Press, 1977), p. 72.

2. Dr. F. Hollick, *The Origin of Life and Process of Reproduction in Plants and Animals, with the Anatomy and Physiology of the Human Generative System, Male and Female, and the Causes, Prevention and Cure of the Special Diseases to which it is Liable. A Plain, Practical Treatise, for Popular Use* (Philadelphia: David McKay, Publisher, 1902), p. 673.

3. Ibid., p. 678.

4. Vern L. Bullough, *Sex, Society and History* (New York: Science History Publications, 1976), p. 173.

5. Quoted in Sarah Stage, *Female Complaints* (New York: W. W. Norton, 1979), p. 90.

6. Ibid., p. 79.

7. Ibid.

8. Ellen Chesler, *Woman of Valor: Margaret Sanger and the Birth Control Movement in America* (New York: Anchor Books, 1992), p. 70.

9. Ibid., p. 68.

10. Ibid., p. 67.

11. Ibid., p. 127.

12. Ibid., p. 84.

13. Bullough, p. 136.

14. Chesler, p. 70.

15. Quoted in Evelyne Berriot-Salvadore, "The Discourse of Medicine and Science." In *A History of Women in the West, Volume 3: Renaissance and Enlightenment Paradoxes*, Georges Duby and Michelle Perrot, eds. (Cambridge: Belknap Press, 1993), p. 360.

16. Wertz and Wertz, p. 105.

17. Quoted in Barbara Ehrenreich and Deidre English, *Complaints and Disorders: The Sexual Politics of Sickness* (New York: Feminist Press, 1973), p. 29.

18. Stage, p. 85.

19. Bullough, p. 136.

20. Gina Corea, *The Hidden Malpractice: How American Medicine Treats Women as Patients and Professionals* (New York: William Morrow and Company, Inc., 1977), p. 90.

21. Quoted in ibid., p. 90.

22. George H. Napheys, *The Physical Life of Women: Advice to the Maiden, Wife and Mother.* Quoted in ibid., p. 91.

23. Carroll Smith-Rosenberg and Charles Rosenberg, "The Female Animal." In *Women and Health in America,* Judith Walzer Leavitt, ed. (Madison: University of Wisconsin Press, 1984), p. 13.

24. Thomas W. Kay, "A Study of Sterility, Its Causes and Treatment" (reprint of 1891 article), *Journal of the American Medical Association* 265, no. 6 (1991): 710.

25. Vern Bullough and Martha Voght, "Women, Menstruation, and Nineteenth-Century Medicine." In *Women and Health in America,* Judith Walzer Leavitt, ed. (Madison: University of Wisconsin Press, 1984), p. 32.

26. Quoted in Ann Dally, *Women under the Knife: A History of Surgery* (New York: Routledge, 1991), p. 89.

27. Jeffrey L. Geller and Linda Harris, *Women of the Asylum* (New York: Anchor, 1994), p. 13.

28. Ibid., p. 15.

29. E. Jarvis, "Causes of Insanity." Quoted in ibid., p. 25.

30. J. McDonald, "Puerperal Insanity." Quoted in ibid., pp. 24–25.

31. E. Jarvis, "Causes of Insanity." Quoted in ibid., p. 25.

32. Ibid.

33. George Rohe, "Lactational Insanity" (reprint of 1893 article), *Journal of the American Medical Association* 270, no. 10 (1993): 1180.

34. Anonymous, "Impairment of the Voice in Female Singers, Due to Diseased Sexual Organs" (reprint of 1892 article), *Journal of the American Medical Association* 268, no. 2 (1992): 37.

35. Ibid.

36. Quoted in Dally, p. 158.

37. Quoted in ibid., pp. 160–64.

38. Hollick, p. 604.

39. Deborah Kuhn McGregor, *Sexual Surgery and the Origins of Gynecology* (New York: Garland, 1989), p. 238.

40. Thomas Szasz, *The Manufacture of Madness* (New York: Harper and Row, 1970), p. 192.

41. Quoted in Vern L. Bullough and Bonnie Bullough, *Sexual Attitudes: Myths and Realities* (Amherst, N.Y.: Prometheus Books, 1995), p. 75.

42. Lois Magner, *The History of Medicine* (New York: Marcel Dekker, 1992), p. 285.

43. Albert Lyons and R. Joseph Petrucelli, *Medicine: An Illustrated History* (New York: Harry N. Abrams, Inc., 1987), p. 529.

44. Quoted in Magner, p. 291.

45. Ibid.

46. James Young Simpson, "Answer to the Religious Objections Advanced Against the Employment of Anaesthetic Agents in Midwifery and Surgery." In *Medicine and Western Civilization,* David Rothman, Steven Marcus, and Stephanie Kiceluk, eds. (New Brunswick, N.J.: Rutgers University Press, 1995), p. 399.

47. Ibid., p. 401.

CHAPTER 8

The Twentieth-Century Uterus

After a scientific and an industrial revolution, one might think that the uterus was safe from interference and free from pain, thanks to two (now acceptable) technologies of modern medicine—anesthesia/analgesia and infection control. But the male medical establishment persisted in its attempts to seize the endometrium regardless of its phase. S. Loewe and F. Lange published their research on steroid hormones and their role in reproductive functions in 1926, but it was not until two years later that B. Zondek identified large amounts of estrogen in the urine of pregnant women.[1] Estrone was isolated by both A. F. Butenandt in Germany and E. A. Doisy in the United States in 1929.[2] Then G. W. Corner and W. M. Allen published "Physiology of the corpus luteum: Production of a special uterine reaction (progestational proliferation) by extracts of the corpus luteum" in the *American Journal of Physiology.* With the identification of these hormones—estrogen and progesterone—menstruation was no longer a mystery. Bleeding was not abnormal;

in technical terms, it resulted from a complex periodic event dependent on alternating flows of estrogen and progesterone. Menses resulted when the functional zone of the endometrium (lining the uterus), after building up for a period of time, sloughed off and shed. It was as simple as that; there was no bad blood or poisonous substance lurking within the uterus.

One might think that this enlightening bit of knowledge would serve to free women from the prison of ancient beliefs, but Western society continued to build its ideological menstrual huts. Taboos with regard to the behavior of menstruating women, both sexual and nonsexual, were still in place. Menstruation continued to be equated with sickness and was not spoken of in polite company. In "A Physician's Counsels to Woman in Health and Disease," Dr. W. C. Taylor wrote:

> We cannot too emphatically urge the importance of regarding these monthly returns as periods of ill health, as days when the ordinary occupations are to be suspended or modified. . . . Long walks, dancing, shopping, riding and parties should be avoided at this time of month invariably and under all circumstances. . . .[3]

And in "Sexual Knowledge," Dr. Winfield Scott Hall advised:

> All heavy exercise should be omitted during the menstrual week . . . a girl should not only retire earlier at this time, but ought to stay out of school from one to three days as the case may be, resting the mind and taking extra hours of rest and sleep.[4]

As will be seen, extreme and obsessive attention to the uterus, as reflected in controversies over birth control, abortion, caesarean section, sterilization, hormone-replacement therapy or hysterectomy at menopause, and the medicalization of pre-menstrual syndrome (PMS), all characterized the twentieth century. Many non-owners of a uterus continued to feel that it was their duty to proclaim their ownership of someone else's uterus. Pregnancy had yet to become a solely private matter of the uterus and its owner. From the bedroom to the birthing room, a male-dominated society continued to exert its political power over the corporeal womb. If a woman wanted to place a physical barrier between her uterus and the flow of spermatic juices—whether that barrier was to be wrapped around her os cervix, syringed into her vagina, or wrapped around her male partner's member—laws made it illegal and religion, immoral.

In the United States, the most outspoken and cogent reformer of the twentieth century was Margaret Sanger. A nurse by profession as well as a tireless champion of reproductive freedom, Sanger was arrested after she published *The Woman Rebel,* a work advocating birth control (Figure 43). Sanger was imprisoned many times and, during one trial, offered the following defense:

> I realize that many . . . cannot sympathize with or countenance the methods I have followed in my attempt to arouse working women to the fact that bringing a child into the world is the greatest responsibility. They tell me that *The Woman Rebel* was badly written; that it was crude; that it was emotional and hysterical; that it mixed issues; that it was defiant, and too radical. Well, to all of these indictments I plead guilty.[5]

In other countries, the uterus had it a bit better. During World War I, government officials in the Netherlands, typically more liberal in their attitudes and aided by a committee of Dutch Neo-Malthusians (those who approved of contraception), analyzed the country in terms of where birth control and OB/GYN information were most conspicuously lacking. They subsequently divided the nation into twenty-four geographic parcels and appointed individuals—many of them nurses—to distribute and fit diaphragms to the women within each sector who needed them.[6] Ellen Chesler writes, "However small this operation, it constituted a substantial health presence in the

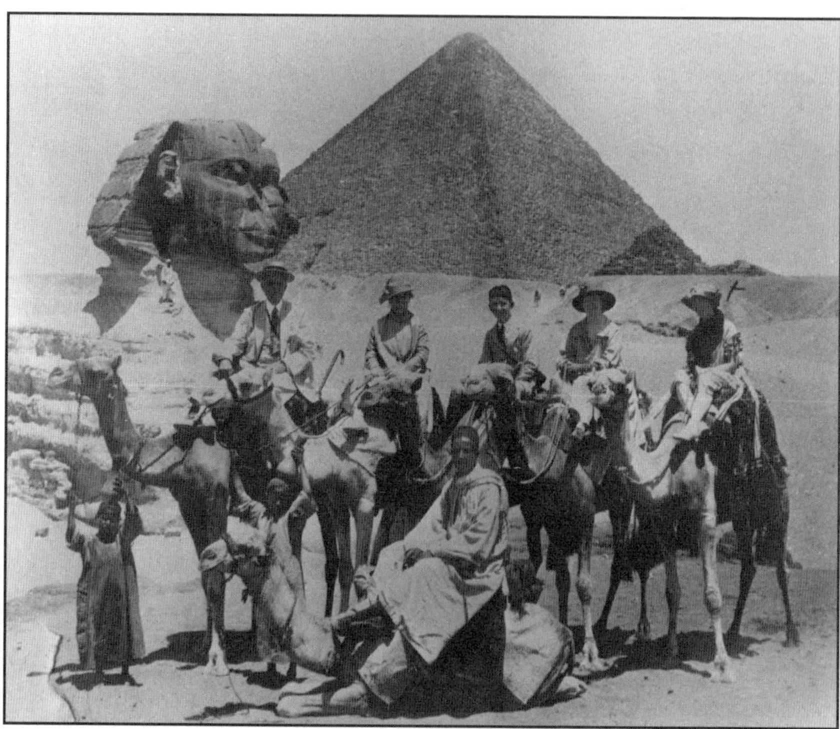

***Figure 43.* Margaret Sanger Goes to Egypt.** After being invited to Japan to lecture on population-control issues, Margaret Sanger traveled to Egypt. She kept a journal and documented cross-cultural birth-control methods. Sanger found that, unlike the ancient Egyptians, those of 1922 no longer employed wax effigies of Thoth. (Sanger is the woman seen "shamelessly" exposing her bare calves). Sophia Smith Collection, Smith College.

gynecological and obstetrical fields and was widely credited for the country's superior maternal and infant mortality statistics."[7]

By World War II, Nazi Germany was advocating other ways to control the uterus. Under the banner of *Kirche, Kinder, und Küche* ("Church, Children, and Kitchen"), the institutionalized scientific racism of the Third Reich sought to control the evolutionary process by unnatural selection. Hitler encouraged the impregnation of every German uterus and offered rewards to those women who had lots of children. A program known as *Lebensborn* encouraged all women who were "racially valuable" to give birth and provided maternity care, child care, and welfare to those who qualified.

In contrast, sterilization courts were set up to hear cases and make decisions on those individuals deemed unfit to reproduce. The first type of sterilization employed was tubal ligation, but Professor G. A. Wagner of the University of Berlin's Women's Clinic

> advocated that the law provide an option for removing the entire uterus in mentally deficient women [because] mentally deficient women, after being sterilized, were especially likely to attract the opposite sex (who need not worry about impregnating them) and therefore to develop gonorrhea . . . the men would then contract gonorrhea from these women . . . and infect other women with desirable hereditary traits and render them sterile.[8]

Finally, after much experimentation, Nazi concentration-camp doctors implemented a program of sterilization by irradiation. They applied such high doses of radiation to Jewish uteruses that the women suffered from external burns and internal tissue necrosis, and they later surgically removed the ovaries just to make certain that germinal material had been ablated.

After World War II, the uterus was allowed to relax a bit. In the United States, the term "family planning" crept into both social and medical vocabularies and it was possible in many states to purchase contraceptive pessaries, condoms, and various spermicides without criminal punishment.

Although an estimated one-third of all American uteri were protected by diaphragms by the 1960s, the method was still not 100 percent reliable.[9] Fortunately, by this time the birth-control pill and the intrauterine device (IUD) were well on their way to becoming the contraceptives of choice, although they, too, had their complications. When the Pill in particular was introduced in 1963, it saved a generation of uteri from the indignities of coat-hanger experiments and unskilled abortionists. The freedom this little steroid brought was unequaled in its repercussions (see Appendix III). Uteri and tubes bounced with joy from Greenwich Village to the Haight, where their owners migrated to dance in parks and protest the Vietnam War. (And not once was the dance equated with hysteria, frenzy, or pathology.) By 1971, far fewer couples used diaphragms. This shift in the choice of contraceptives was fortunate because in May 1977, eighty-six thousand Koro-Flex shields were recalled from use because 1 percent of them had pinprick-sized holes along the rim.[10] Had this diaphragm defect occurred before the Pill was invented, the repercussions would have been drastically more serious.

Changes in law were coming as well. When Jane Roe's uterus failed to proliferate and shed its endometrium in 1972, Roe knew that she was pregnant again and didn't want to go through nine months of changes. Two lawyers agreed that women like Roe who did not want to be pregnant (and already were) have the right to privacy and to legally abort the product of their conception. Of course, this created a new round of social unrest because it meant that women wanted to gain control over their own bodies and this went against tradition. But Jane Roe's lawyers persisted and, on January 22, 1973, the U.S. Supreme Court handed down this historic decision:

> The right of privacy is broad enough to encompass a woman's decision whether or not to terminate her pregnancy. . . . Only a pregnant woman and her doctor have the right to make the decision about an abortion.[11]

Now that birth control and abortion are legal, other issues confront the uterus. One of them is class difference. For example, upper- and middle-class women prefer to limit the size of their families for a variety of personal and professional reasons. Many working-class and ethnic-minority women, on the other hand, positively value a large family and repeated impregnation of the uterus. Legislators now want to control the wombs of these latter groups because they feel that the state will ultimately be responsible for the care and feeding of any children these people may have. As a consequence, a number of political and even coercive measures have been developed in order to discourage a high birth rate among these groups. One unique birth-control device, Norplant, has been used as a subcutaneous implant that releases regular doses of an anti-ovulation hormone over a period of time. This automatic trickle precludes the hormone's not being taken regularly due to forgetfulness or a financial or logistical inability to refill the prescription several times a year. The release of the hormone lasts approximately five years, but the implant has to be inserted and replaced by a physician. Despite the advantages of Norplant and similar methods, their use among certain predictable groups—the working poor, welfare recipients, and black and Latino women—sends a message that is distressingly clear: We want you to control the proliferation of "your kind," but not the same way "we" do—an implicitly racist agenda.

When the uterus slows its cycle of shedding the endometrium, perimenopause is said to begin. This process, about ten years in all, is gradual and accompanied by "hysteria" only in the last two or three years—and then in only about 40 percent of women. But "the Change" is not only dreaded, it carries with it a societal stigma. As Paula Weideger notes, "The more avidly one embraces the belief that motherhood is holy and fertility golden, the greater the conviction that menopause is the corrosive end to all that is desirable and worthwhile."[12]

One popular treatment for menopause is hysterectomy. A typical scenario is described in Gail Sheehy's book, *The Silent*

Passage: "A woman who is perimenopausal but doesn't know it goes to her doctor to report heavy bleeding. 'Is this the Change?' she asks. He tells her she is too young for the Change but she'd better have a D&C. . . ."[13] But the heavy bleeding does not stop because it is normal, although this fact is often simply not mentioned to the distressed patient. When the woman returns to the doctor, she is told to have another D&C and then another. When the second or third try is equally unsuccessful, the doctor convinces her that she needs a hysterectomy. With the surgical removal of the uterus, the women's menopause is now complete. Her body has bypassed the normal process of gradual change over a ten-year period in just one or two. Menopause, like menstruation and childbirth, has now been medicalized, the modern way to signal a rite of passage. But this "progress" hasn't come without a price. Since ovariotomy (removal of the ovaries) is routinely done at the time of the hysterectomy (called TAH/BSO, total abdominal hysterectomy and bilateral salpingooophorectomy), the woman's hot flashes are immediate and severe. Surgical menopause, unlike biological menopause, is intense and immediate, without respite. Unless the woman is given HRT (hormone-replacement therapy) estrogen, her bone density will be lost at a greater rate than normal. The vaginal mucosa will thin, making intercourse uncomfortable or painful.

Even the rhetoric that accompanies the discussion of a possible hysterectomy in a perimenopausal woman is revealing, especially with regard to the power and knowledge differential that the doctor-patient relationship typically demonstrates. The patient (the owner of the body and uterus) asks the doctor (the keeper of the power and knowledge) why a hysterectomy has been advised. The doctor responds, "Your uterus looks a little tired." Or, "You don't need it any more." Or, "Why would you want a uterus if you're not going to have any more children?" Or, "You will never have to be inconvenienced by bleeding again." Such language suggests that the uterus has a personality of its own, or that it has no use unless it is going to be impregnated. It also omits the obvious—that the inconvenience of bleeding will stop on its own quite soon, without any intervention. The language of menopause is consistent with the pejorative tone of medical language throughout most of female history. Ovarian "failure," rather than "retirement" or "closure," is used to describe the reason why the cessation of menses occurs (Figure 44).

At least we have graduated from the earlier paradigm of female suffering as the punishment of God for Eve's disobedience. One hundred years ago, eugenicists B. G. Jeffries and J. L. Nichols, in their book *Safe Counsel, or Practical Eugenics,* described "temporary mental derangement [as] one of the most common symptoms of the menopause. . . . This may last for a few weeks only, or it may drag along for years."[14] And barely fifty years ago, the authors of *The Illustrated Encyclopedia of Sex* wrote that the itching of the genital organs

> manifests itself in almost unbearable irritation and burning . . . frequently accompanied with libidinous sensations, which may be so intense that unless relief can be obtained through conjugal intercourse, excessive masturbation may be resorted to. Dr. Magnus Hirschfeld in his *Sexual Pathology* records the cases of women who were driven to nymphomania as the result of this tormenting irritation.[15]

One wonders what happened to those women who had to "resort" to "excessive masturbation"—did they survive? And what of the nymphomaniacs? More to the point, has the nature of menopause changed, or our ways of understanding it? When woman's only value to society is her role as child bearer, it is only logical that she will mourn the loss of this function. Likewise, if she is not allowed to scratch an itch or relieve her sexual feelings though an acceptable avenue of satisfaction, her frustration will be overt. How ironic, too, that the current physiological characterizations of menopause—*hot* flashes and vaginal *dryness*—are exactly the opposite of those humoral qualities of

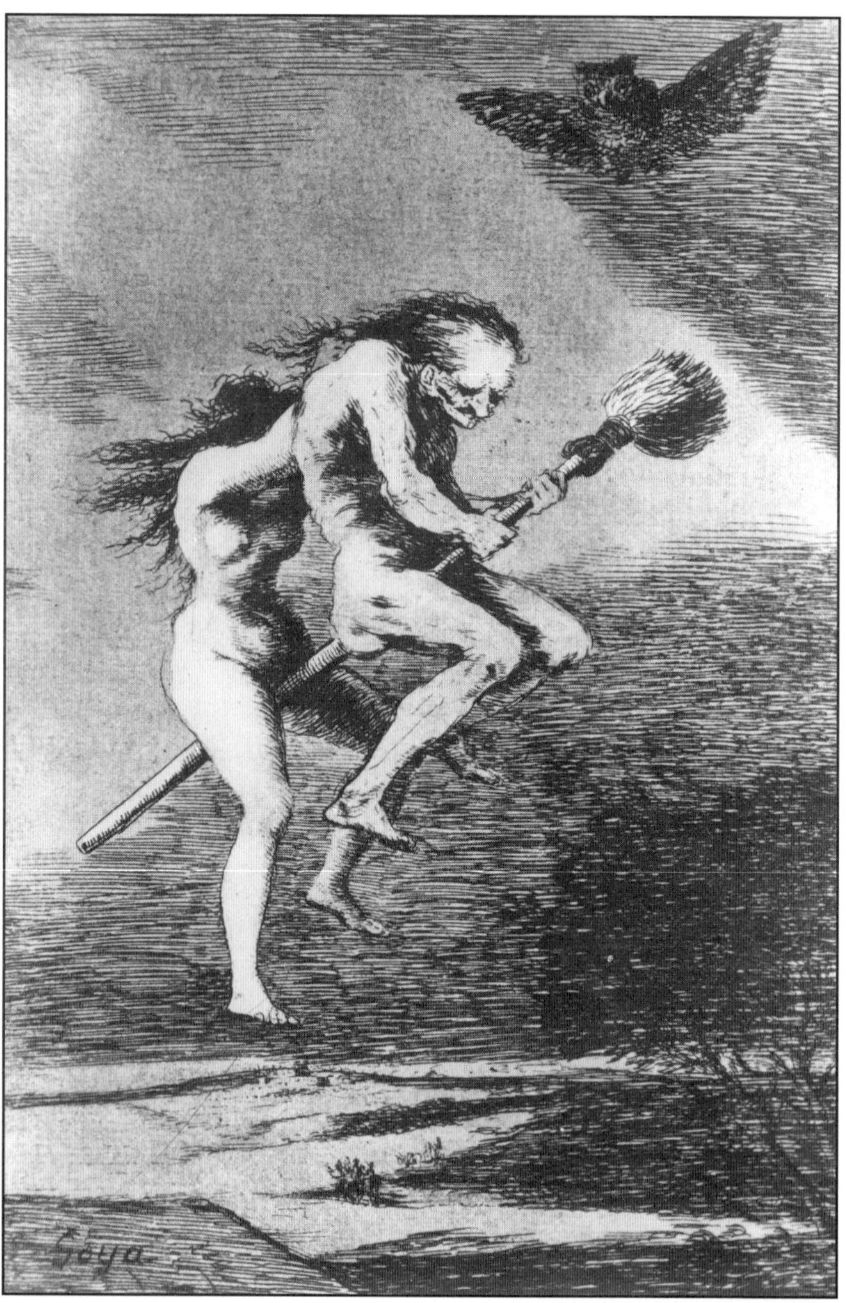

Francisco de Goya y Lucientes. Plate 68 from "Los Caprichos": Linda maestra (attractive master). Courtesy: FOTO Marburg/Art Resource, New York.

***Figure 44.* A Witch's Image and the Postmenopausal Woman.** The witch and the postmenopausal woman have much in common. Tooth loss results in diminished vertical height of the face. The lips are no longer supported by the teeth and the facial expression is dour. Osteoporosis in the cervical and thoracic areas of the spine causes loss of height in the neck vertebrae. Small compression fractures cause the characteristic "dowager's hump" seen in so many older women and images of witches. Subsequent compression fractures in the thoracic area cause an AP kyphosis or "hunchback." When osteoarthritis affects the lumbar area, a person has difficulty walking and may limp or have to use a cane. Vocal-cord changes due to stridor cause jerky phonation and scratchy speech. Both the witch and the postmenopausal woman have sagging breasts and other physical changes such as hair loss.

Witches were often associated with nature, lush greenery, fertility, growth and rebirth, and sexuality. As the philosophy of religion evolved, they were blamed for male impotence, identified as the cause of adultery, and said to possess insatiable sexual hungers which no mortal man could satisfy. Perhaps the idea of a sexy, desirable witch was too dangerous to court. Many fine-art images of the witch show an ugly, undesirable, older woman. The association of "witch" with "older woman" is demonstrated in our use of the word "hag," meaning an evil female spirit, "crone," a withered old woman, or "crow," the symbol for the death-goddess (or valkyrie).

---

females (i.e., cold and moist). Medicalization offers hormone-replacement therapy to make women cold and moist once again, but not all women seek this kind of resolution. For some, this passage leads to a new world of nonreproductive, nonbiological values, where anatomy is not destiny and where new kinds of achievement are possible.

As the twentieth century draws to a close, women's health issues are dependent on a variety of curious technologies. Embedded in popular culture, these medical choices, like the Sorcerer's Apprentice, create more of themselves, flooding the gates of the imagination. Reproduction can now be controlled with chemicals in young women and with tubal ligation in those who choose permanent sterility. Even those who request "natural childbirth" may have to submit to a very unnatural fetal monitor at some point; they still labor within a medicalized set of parameters, however invisible they may be at the moment. Likewise, if labor contractions prove too painful, they can be eased with laughing gas, an epidural block, or a combination of safe analgesics. As Judith Walzer Leavitt points out in "Birthing and Anesthesia: The Debate over Twilight Sleep," in the early years of the twentieth century women felt that with the use of scopolamine and morphine, they would gain control over the birthing process (even though it meant going to sleep). According to Leavitt, problems arose because the control women wanted was control without physicians and, "in the face of advancing obstetrical technology, many physicians wanted to retain their professional right and duty to decide therapy on the basis of their judgment . . . they refused to be 'dragooned' into 'indiscriminate adoption' of a procedure that they themselves did not choose."[16] Leavitt argues that, far from increasing women's control, the imposition of "twilight sleep" distanced women from their own bodies.

What appears to be a paradox with regard to the use of morphine and scopolamine is also evident in the diversity of attitudes with regard to caesarean section. Many women who have undergone c-section feel that they had more control over the birth because they were able to watch the entire experience. Others point out that control rests with the decision-maker and, since it is the doctor who decides if and when a caesarean is necessary, the women in fact had no control. Then, too, from an evolutionary standpoint, natural selection for a large pelvic outlet is no longer taking place as a result of so many caesarean sections. On the other hand, there are undoubtedly thousands of women every year who, without a caesarean section, might have died in childbirth due to the complications arising from a fetal head too big to pass through the pubic arch.

One could argue, in fact, that with the use of chemical, mechanical, and surgical methods to alter uterine physiology, nature has been trumped by technology. It remains to future theorists to analyze the Darwinian effects of these changes. We embrace technology to enhance our lives but, in doing so, lose a certain amount of shared cultural information about our bodies.

The risk is that we may become passive recipients of medicalized culture—and the more technology is promoted, the less choice we actually have because doctors control the technology. Even this would be more acceptable if physician education was not steeped in centuries of mythology about menstrual pollution, uncontrollable sexuality, and value based on biological fecundity.

ENDNOTES

1. Ferid Murad and Robert C. Haynes Jr., "Estrogens and Progestins." In Louis S. Goodman and Alfred Gilman, *The Pharmacological Basis of Therapeutics* (New York: Macmillan, 1985), p. 1412.

2. Bernard Grun, *The Timetables of History* (New York: Simon and Schuster, 1991), p. 497.

3. W. C. Taylor, "A Physician's Counsels to Woman in Health and Disease." Quoted in Barbara Ehrenreich and Deidre English, *For Her Own Good* (New York: Anchor Books, 1978), p. 111.

4. Winfield Scott Hall, "Sexual Knowledge." Quoted in Ehrenreich and English, p. 111.

5. Quoted in Ellen Chesler, *Woman of Valor: Margaret Sanger and the Birth Control Movement in America* (New York: Anchor Books, 1992), p. 140.

6. Chesler, p. 146.

7. Ibid.

8. Quoted in Robert Jay Lifton, *The Nazi Doctors: Medical Killing and the Psychology of Genocide* (New York: Basic Books, 1986), p. 26.

9. The Boston Women's Health Collective, *The New Our Bodies, Ourselves* (New York: Touchstone, 1984), p. 225.

10. Ibid.

11. Ibid., p. 311.

12. Paula Weideger, *Menstruation and Menopause* (New York: Alfred A. Knopf, 1976), p. 197.

13. Gail Sheehy, *The Silent Passage* (New York: Pocket Books, 1993), p. 65.

14. B. G. Jeffries and J. L. Nichols, *Safe Counsel, or Practical Eugenics* (New York: Intext Press, 1928), p. 195.

15. Dr. A. Willy, Dr. L. Vander, Dr. O. Fisher, et al., *The Illustrated Encyclopedia of Sex* (N.p.: Royton Publishing Co., 1977), p. 374.

16. Judith Walzer Leavitt, "Birthing and Anesthesia: The Debate over Twilight Sleep." In *Women and Health in America*, Judith Walzer Leavitt, ed. (Madison: University of Wisconsin Press, 1984), pp. 180–81.

CHAPTER 9

The Postmodern Uterus

I found myself last night thinking about the day and the Cesarean I had done. Performing a Cesarean is the one time that truly gives you the feeling of delivering the baby. I remember having my hand in the uterus. Pressure was being applied by Dr. Joseph at the top of the uterus while my hand grasped the head of the baby and assisted it out through the incision. I felt a sense of excitement and of power and of personal accomplishment that is not present in a vaginal birth. This is the time the obstetrician truly delivers the baby; in a vaginal birth, it is the mother.

—Michelle Harrison, "A Woman in Residence"[1]

In *Brave New World,* written in 1931, Aldous Huxley transported his readers six hundred years into the future, where one egg and one sperm would form an embryo in a test tube that would produce ninety-six human beings—the principle of mass production applied to biology. Society was produced in groups of Alphas, Betas, Gammas, Deltas, and Epsilons, each group with a predetermined level of intelligence. Pavlovian conditioning was used to control the behavior of each group, providing stimulus-

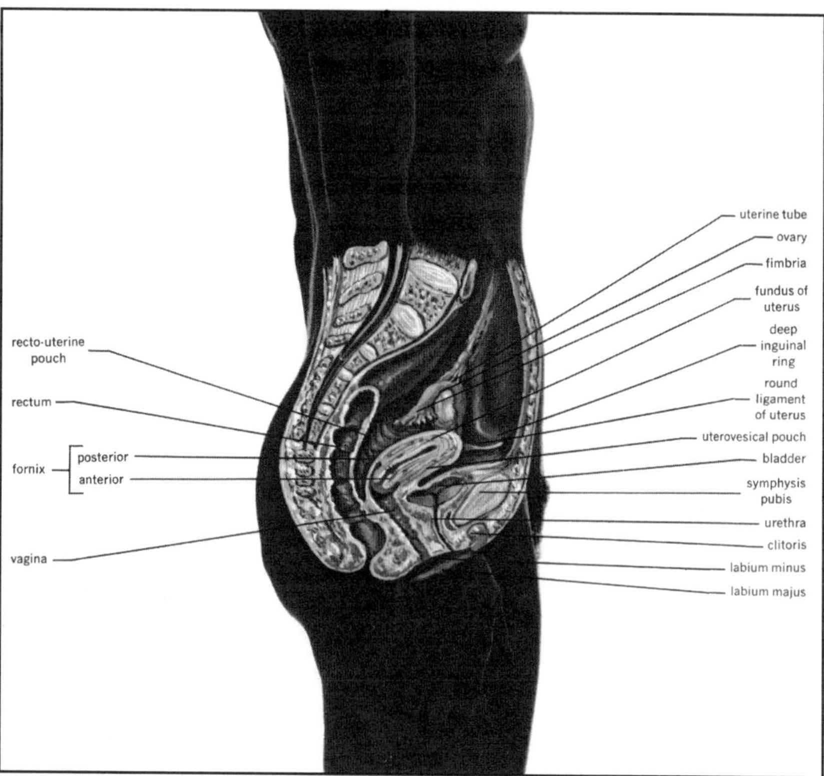

Figure 45. **The Stilled Uterus.** The uterus is no longer an animal within an animal. It has gone from being a structural entity that travels through the body with a will of its own to a stable (albeit passive) system located within the pelvic cavity. In 1980, Alvin Silverstein, author of *Human Anatomy and Physiology,* wrote, "It seems extraordinary that a 7- or 8-pound human infant . . . can be accommodated inside an organ that, in its normal nonpregnant state, is no bigger than a small pear." A few years later, the authors of *Principles of Anatomy and Physiology,* Gerald Tortera, Gerald Anagnostakos, and Nicholas Anagnostakos, described the uterus as "the site of menstruation, implantation of a fertilized ovum, development of the fetus during pregnancy, and labor. . . ." In 1992, Frederic Martini described it in *Fundamentals of Anatomy and Physiology* with a single sentence: "The uterus provides mechanical protection and nutritional support to the developing embryo." These limited descriptions offer clues as to why physicians advise women who are beyond childbearing to get rid of their uterus because they no longer "need" it.

response situations to either reinforce for or sensitize against certain behaviors. At one point in the novel, the resident controller shouts, "Try to remember what it was like to have a viviparous mother," but no one can. By that time—the year A.F. 632—there is no use for the uterus.

At the close of the twentieth century, the uterus has traveled from the pelvis to the brain and back again (Figure 45). The ancient concept "suffocation of the mother" has been replaced by some equally strange terms: An *incompetent cervix* is one that opens prematurely during pregnancy; *ovarian failure* is another term for menopause; and *ovarian fibrillations* (not a real medical term) is a vernacular diagnosis for behaviors that doctors can't medicalize. Even today, if a man and a woman with similar medical histories go to an emergency room with chest pains, the woman is more likely than the man to be given a psychogenic diagnosis and to be questioned about her reproductive status and sexual history.

Doctors used to blame pathologic muscular movements of the abdomen as a cause of interference with the laboring uterus. Its sequelae reportedly caused the toxemia of pregnancy. The theory behind these ideas is that the female body rebels against a parturient uterus with the same vengeance with which it repels a foreign protein. In the words of Robert T. Francoeur:

> A woman's uterus pushes forward and changes in shape from oval to near spherical. The tensed muscles of the abdomen often interfere with this transformation, causing pain and prolonging the birth. The rather general assumption has been that toxemia and the convulsions it brings on are due to the increasing pressures of the abdominal muscles reducing the flow of blood in the uterus and placenta.[2]

To assist in relief from the problems associated with toxic pregnancies, a variety of remedies were offered. The pregnancy was viewed as invasive and abnormal, so help was directed at reducing physiological pressures. Hence, the "Birthezz": a body suit with a fiberglass dome over the abdomen. The user would change the atmospheric pressure inside her uterus by connecting the dome to a vacuum cleaner, decompressing the suit. Decompressions were performed three times a week for twenty minutes each. The results were documented in glowing terms by the inventor, Dr. Ockert Heyns. His rationale was that in the final trimester of pregnancy, the fetus grows faster than the placenta, which means that its heart cannot pump as easily as before. By making the uterus superoxygenated, babies who were in utero had not only improved cardiac function but also increased IQ scores. Heyns's claims were never thoroughly verified. Regardless of their accuracy, however, the Birthezz is an early example of the attempt to change the uterine environment in order to influence or affect the future individual's behavior (see Appendix IV).

Fiberglass domes were only the beginning of a trend that has focused more on the baby than the mother, the end result being that the uterus (an organ) takes supremacy over its owner (the person). Intrauterine television, for example, has given us glimpses of a swimming, exercising fetus that can feel pain. The unpredicted consequence of this invasion of somatic privacy is to set back still further the boundaries of "personhood." This concept—so crucial to recent abortion-rights debates—is culturally variable, ranging from a broad Confucian interpretation that extends into family and social circle to an extremely narrow interpretation that puts the locus of "life" at the moment of fertilization.

"Viability" is an ambiguous concept as well. Once the quickening that occurs at approximately five months was thought to define the onset of life. More recently, the stethoscope amplified the fetal heartbeat and extended life backward one or two months. When fiber optics were added to the imaging toolkit, an early embryo could actually be observed in utero (Figure 46). The TV monitor with its grainy ultrasound images can now be employed to show the configurations of a primitive spinal cord, even to the point of diagnosing abnormalities. At one time, "baby pictures" were prints developed from film exposed soon after the baby emerged into the non-

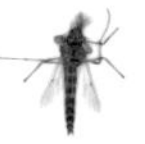

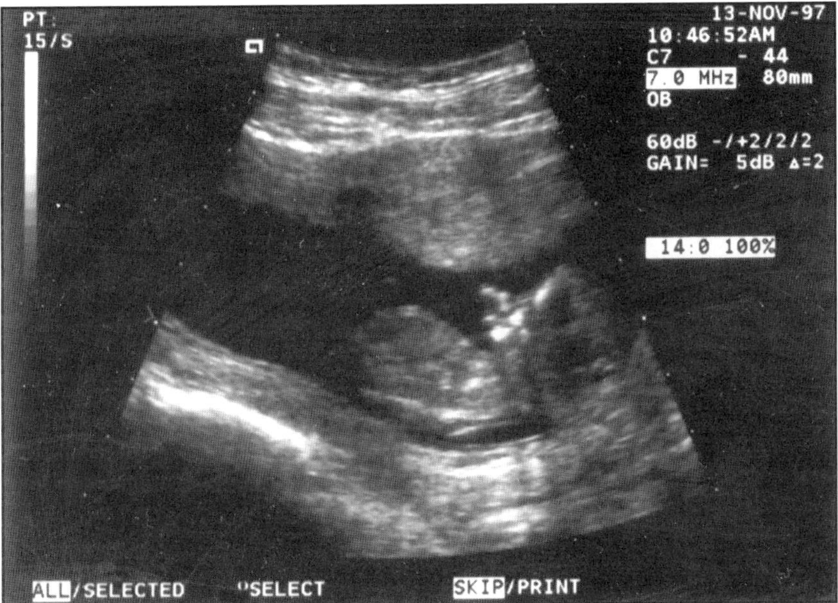

***Figure 46.* The Postmodern Fetus.** Unlike the medieval product of conception—floating in an ocean of amniotic fluid, evidently conscious and looking outward, ready to emerge fully formed into the world—the ultrasound fetus remains naively unaware of any invasion of privacy. The ultrasound image can reveal many uterine abnormalities, such as anencephaly, an empty gestational sac, or fibroid tumors. The sex of the child is apparent by three months and precludes the necessity of a more invasive procedure.

Author Robbie Davis-Floyd sees ultrasonography as just one more step in the process of technocratic childbirth, from amniocentesis to fetal monitor, to induced labor with pitocin, epidural anesthesia, caesarean section, a doctor's gloved hands, a nurse's inspection, silver nitrate drops in the eyes, bottle-feeding, and caregivers in a nursery rather than the mother.

uterine environment. These days, they are likely to be a sequence of ultrasound images with the baby floating in amniotic fluid—our own version of the little man pictured inside the pre-Renaissance uterus. Look closely the next time someone offers to show you such pictures—he or she has automatically accepted the retro-boundary of life and considers these sequenced ultrasound images synonymous with personhood. Humankind shares an interest in the mysterious uterine world, and ultrasound techniques have changed to keep up with the demand for more information about prenatal life. In 1996, the Food and Drug Administration approved Toshiba's Eccocee, an $85,000 color-image system. The latest machines are digital and show clearer pictures than the older analog models.

Ironically, now that life can be imaged as far back as the first few weeks, the moral implications of sustaining that life are more complex than medieval debates about when the soul entered the body. As Margaret Clark observes, "In western society today, the crux of the abortion controversy lies in the ambiguity about the definition of a person at the beginning of life. . . . There is no question that medical technology has influenced some of these beliefs."[3] In cultures that value male over female life and allow only one child per family, an ultrasound can be used to justify either the destruction or the preservation of a new life based entirely on sex. Hiroshi Nakajima, Director General of the World Health Organization, writes that "discrimination begins for women while they are still in the womb: the desirability of a male child is still unquestioned in many societies, prompting families to abort female fetuses or to abandon or even murder them at birth."[4]

For a brief period in the history of the uterus, *Roe* v. *Wade* improved the safety and viability of the newly pregnant woman. Recently, there has been a backlash self-proclaimed do-gooders who, in defending the contents of the uterus as having a "right to life," have severely compromised the uterus owner. Just when the uterus was breathing a sigh of relief from all the political clatter, religious fanatics, shouting that abortion was murder, gunned down the gatekeepers of family-planning clinics and the physicians who performed the procedure. These self-righteous, Bible-spewing bigots use language laced with terms like *evil* and *sin* as they seek to devalue and objectify women once again, returning them to the status of receptacles or vessels. Those who spread their ignorance regarding women as incubators for the growth of the "unborn" appear to share pre-scientific ideas about the *homunculus* ("little man")—that it is he, within the womb, who initiates labor and controls his birth, and not anything or anyone else.

It's not just abortions that are under scrutiny, but the methods of childbirth as well. According to William Curran in the *New England Journal of Medicine,* "In a quiet, often unnoticed, but consistent manner, a number of trial-court judges in at least 11 states across the country have ordered that a pregnant woman just submit to a cesarean section to deliver a viable fetus against the known and clearly expressed will of the woman."[5] These women have been Hispanic, black, or Asian, did not speak English as a primary language, or else belonged to families that held alternative healing beliefs foreign to the U.S. biomedical system. Thus the provisions of *Roe* v. *Wade* have been turned upside down; conservative judges now insist that "once the woman makes the decision early in the pregnancy about whether to carry the fetus to term, she has a legal obligation to protect" its safety and health.[6] Fortunately, the U.S. Court of Appeals re-examined the decision in one of these cases and pointed out that *Roe* v. *Wade* never gave the fetus primary or equal status with the pregnant woman. By overturning the lower court's decision, the appeals court provided strong support for the primacy of the woman's rights when they are threatened by procedures to protect the fetus. As William Curran noted in conclusion, "In my judgment, the decision in this case turns the law in the proper direction."[7]

Every function of the uterus can now be studied and controlled, from menarche to menopause. If Augustine were able to spend some time in our century, he would be amazed. Not only can the procreative act be performed without passion or pleasure (as he advocated), but the uterus can now sustain a product of conception without sexual intercourse. Indeed, by the 1980s, experiments had proved that the uterus was not essential for fertilization. In this brave new world, cold Petri dishes can house zygotes of unknown origin until they exceed their media. Then a uterus (any uterus) can be used to foster the growth of an egg (any egg) that has been fertilized by a sperm (any sperm). In one recent case, a sixty-three-year-old woman long past her fertile years offered to house her daughter's embryo in her own uterus until it was full-term. Although the uterus is not discriminatory, this situation presents many problems for clergy and laiety alike. In one bizarre miscarriage of postmodern technology, a doctor who operated a fertility clinic in Vienna, Virginia, was found to have used his own sperm to inseminate women whose husbands were unable to father children. (His lawyer defended him by saying that "he was a qualified donor in a time when there is much disease about.") "Dr. J." extracted his sperm in the privacy of his office bathroom shortly before the arrival of each patient, later telling them he had located a donor after an extensive search.

In *Birth as an American Rite of Passage,* Robbie E. Davis-Floyd argues that the uterus has become medicalized to the point that women are hardly in touch with the process of childbearing. The parturient woman's uterus is watched on an ultrasound screen. Sometimes pitocin, a powerful hormone, is administered intravenously so that the baby can be delivered at a time most convenient to either the executive mom's work schedule or the doctor's golf game, vacation, or required hours of sleep. Often a caesarian is planned so that a birth will not conflict with another family event, and sometimes so it will coincide with another. (For example, a mother might want her child to be born on St. Valentine's Day or Rosh Hashanah.) We are even at a point where futurists imagine a scenario in which a fertilized ovum implanted in the peritoneal cavity of a male will grow to viability and then be removed via caesarion (a male caesarean).

Throughout her book, Davis-Floyd argues that the hospital as an institution has removed power, privacy, and choice from the patient. She calls this model *technocratic,* the "etic view." She also informs the reader that many of the women who have undergone this postmodern rite of passage do not feel that they have been cheated out of *experience,* the "emic view."[8] Many feminists, aware of both views, promote a return to the midwife-attended birth; and true to the culture of institutions, some hospitals now "allow" midwives to come through their doors as practitioners, provided they are licensed and associated with a medical practice. This policy varies from state to state, but the point is that technocracy wins by incorporating the services of one more "specialist." There are also some "birthing centers" that employ only midwives and some midwife attendance at home births as well, but it is doubtful that midwives will practice as autonomously as they once did, even with more formal medical education. All too often, they must still be connected by some official link to a medical institution.

❖ ❖ ❖

The postmodern uterus is entitled to both appropriate ownership and maintenance. It is no longer sufficient to tell a woman that she needn't worry her pretty little head over her own body. She must be prepared to navigate that body through an intricate and highly complex network of ideas and attitudes in order to reach a resolution of the problem.

If a woman is insistent and persistent enough, she can demand to be fully informed about any suggested procedure relating to her uterus. This does not guarantee a lack of defensive posture on the part of the physician if the patient "asks too many questions" (Figure 47). When the Public Citizen Health Research Group did a study on caesarean births, it found that in 1992, "420,000 unnecessary c-sections were performed."[9] The normal expected proportion of birth by caesarean section is 12 percent, and this number represented an overall c-section rate

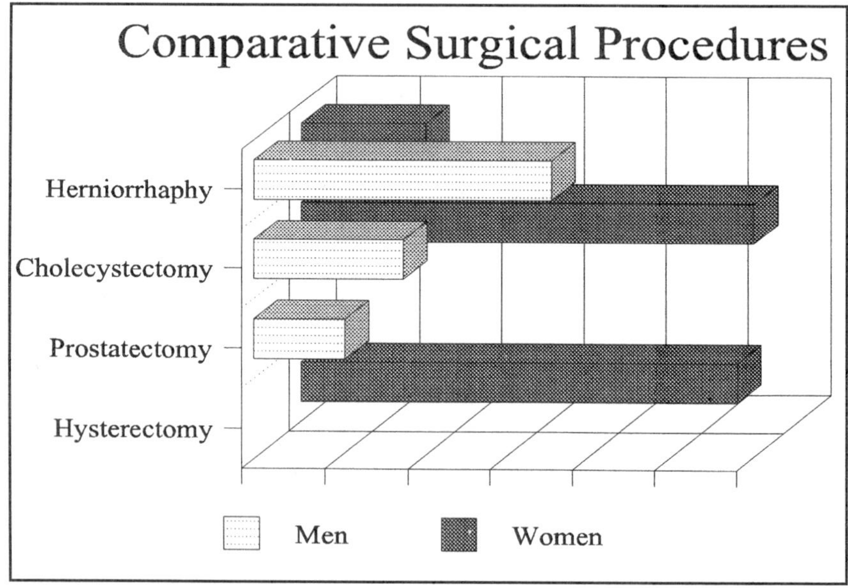

Figure 47. **Informed Consent Needed.** Many women report that their questions in this culture of hysterectomies are not answered. They feel they lack the necessary information to make an informed decision. Some critics point out that physicians prefer to own the knowledge about gynecology, perhaps because they benefit financially from the surgeries. Hysterectomies rank second only to c-sections among the most common surgeries performed on women, according to a *New York Times* article in February 1997. In a 1993 report by the subcommittee on aging, Vivian W. Pinn, M.D., found that the number of hysterectomies peaked in 1975 at 740,000. That same report also stated that by the age of 60, 35 percent of American women will have had a hysterectomy. Death rates from this procedure range from 6 to 11 per 10,000, with nonfatal complications in 25 to 50 percent of the cases. In comparison with other, similar surgeries performed on either men or women—prostatectomy (removal of the prostate), hysterectomy (removal of the uterus), cholecystectomy (gall bladder removal), and herniorraphy (hernia repair)—hysterectomy ranked first.

of 22.6 percent. Interestingly, the highest rates were in the South and at for-profit hospitals; Arkansas had the highest rate (28.4 percent) and Colorado the lowest (16.3 percent). Since hysterectomies and c-sections are two of the most common surgeries recommended to women, those who are considering these operations would do well to read up on them if their doctors do not answer their questions satisfactorily. And as more women graduate from medical schools and enter into the fields of obstetrics and gynecology, it will be useful to see if these procedures are recommended by them to the same degree as by their male colleagues. (It may turn out that the penchant to do surgery is related more to financial gain than to gender).

This book was written to make people, particularly female people, aware of the tremendous social, psychological, religious, and medical pressures brought to bear upon the uterus as it traveled through history. My intention in writing this book was to help women recognize the specious and faulty thinking they have been the targets of throughout history, as demonstrated by the concept of hysteria and all the other syndromes attributed to their "inferior bodies"and "wandering wombs."

The research I did for this book was an immensely valuable experience. It showed me how an old idea can remain embedded in a culture if no one comes along to challenge it. The history of medicine is filled with myths about the human body as well as many insufficient medical paradigms, from those that used pigs as the model for the female reproductive system to those that conceive of human beings as the product of medical institutions. These are the ideological pillars that support how women are perceived and treated. If a diagnosis does not make sense to you, don't consent to surgery until you are satisfied that you know all your options. Information is widely available, and medical journal abstracts can be accessed on the Internet. It's more than a second opinion, it's the entire world of opinion. Read up on the advice you've been given. (If you don't own a computer, most libraries have one or more for public use.) For centuries, male doctors have aligned themselves with a male god to the detriment of their female patients. It's difficult to change that attitude.

Just as this book was going to press, the staid, conservative *Journal of the American Medical Association* published an entire issue on "alternative medicine." In this November 11, 1998, issue was an article about the use of moxibustion to turn fetuses to cephalic presentation that are currently in breech positions. Moxibustion, used in the People's Republic of China, is an ancient technique of burning herbs to stimulate acupuncture points. This particular point is called *Zhiyin,* located beside the outside corner of the fifth toenail. The group studied received two half-hour stimulations per day and reportedly showed a "significant increase in cephalic version within two weeks of the start of therapy and in cephalic presentations at birth." The Chinese researchers reported that the effect of burning herbs is on maternal plasma cortisol and post-glandins, but the authors of the *JAMA* article note that the "mechanism of action of moxibustion is not entirely clear and warrants further research." It is interesting that, after coming more than eight thousand years in two hundred pages from early notions of aromatherapy as a treatment for the wandering womb, we should arrive at a point where a similar and equally mysterious treatment would capture the attention of a medical journal editor. How fitting for the postmodern uterus.

To conclude, I'd like to propose a thought experiment. Try to imagine how different women's history would have been if the Bible had stated that man was created from the rib of a woman, that Adam tempted Eve with forbidden fruit and got them expelled from paradise, and that Eve's body was the ideal and Adam's the anomaly. What if, allegedly as a result of Adam's original sin, men were doomed to suffer from a sharp pain in the prostate each time they impregnated a woman, and when they went to a urologist to find some relief, they were told that their suffering was God's will? Additionally, what if, because they ejaculated and produced a sticky, salty fluid, they were thought to be warlocks? Think how traumatic it would have been for a male child to produce this strange substance after a dream and then be hauled off before the Grand Inquisitor as a result. What if an entire cult had spread over Europe torturing and executing any man who produced this strange fluid after his prostate was massaged, and two nuns had written a book that explained how to recognize this warlockian behavior? And what if his medical care was focused exclusively on his prostate because it was considered the cause of all his illness—or if, when he complained of a musculoskeletal pain, he was told that it was just "male trouble"? What if only women were educated and men were not allowed to go to school because brainwork would take away from their reproductive power, and men were made to reproduce, not to study? What if only women could be heads of state, doctors, lawyers, judges, or any other high-paying and powerful profession, and men could only be secretaries and houseworkers because they might damage their prostates?

If all that seems odd or ridiculous, then you have benefited from our brief survey of the wandering womb, a cultural history of outrageous beliefs about women.

ENDNOTES

1. Michelle Harrison, "A Woman in Residence." Quoted in Robbie Davis-Floyd, *Birth as an American Rite of Passage* (Berkeley: University of California Press, 1992), p. 130.
2. Robert T. Francoeur, *Utopian Motherhood: New Trends in Human Reproduction* (New York: Doubleday, 1970), p. 164.
3. Margaret Clark, "Medical Anthropology and the Redefining of Human Nature," *Human Organization* 52, no. 3 (1993): 235.
4. Quoted in Marianne J. Legato, "Tomorrow the World," *The Female Patient* (April 1996): 15.
5. William J. Curran, "Court Ordered Caesarean Sections Receive Judicial Defeat," *New England Journal of Medicine* 323, no. 7 (1990): 489.
6. Ibid.
7. Ibid.
8. Davis-Floyd, p. 281.
9. "420,000 C-Sections a Year Are Called Unneeded," *New York Times* (May 22, 1994), p. 30.

APPENDIX I

On Difficult Labor

Paul of Aegina (632–690 C.E.)*

Difficult labour arises either from the woman who bears the child, or from the child itself, or from the secundines, or from some external circumstances. From the woman in labour, either because she is gross and fat, or because her whole womb is small, or because she has no pains, or is affected with fear, or because the uterus or some other part is inflamed or otherwise weakened, or because from some natural weakness, she is unable to expel the foetus, or because the labour is premature. From the child, either because it is too large; or small, and of little weight; or from its having hydrocephalous head; or from being a monster, such as having two heads; or because it is dead; or, although alive, because it is weak and unable to advance outward; or because there happens to be several children, as Herophilus relates a case of five; or because the position is preternatural. For the natural position of

*From Herbert Thoms, *Classical Contributions to Obstetrics and Gynecology* (Springfield, Ill.: Charles C Thomas, 1935). Courtesy of the publisher.

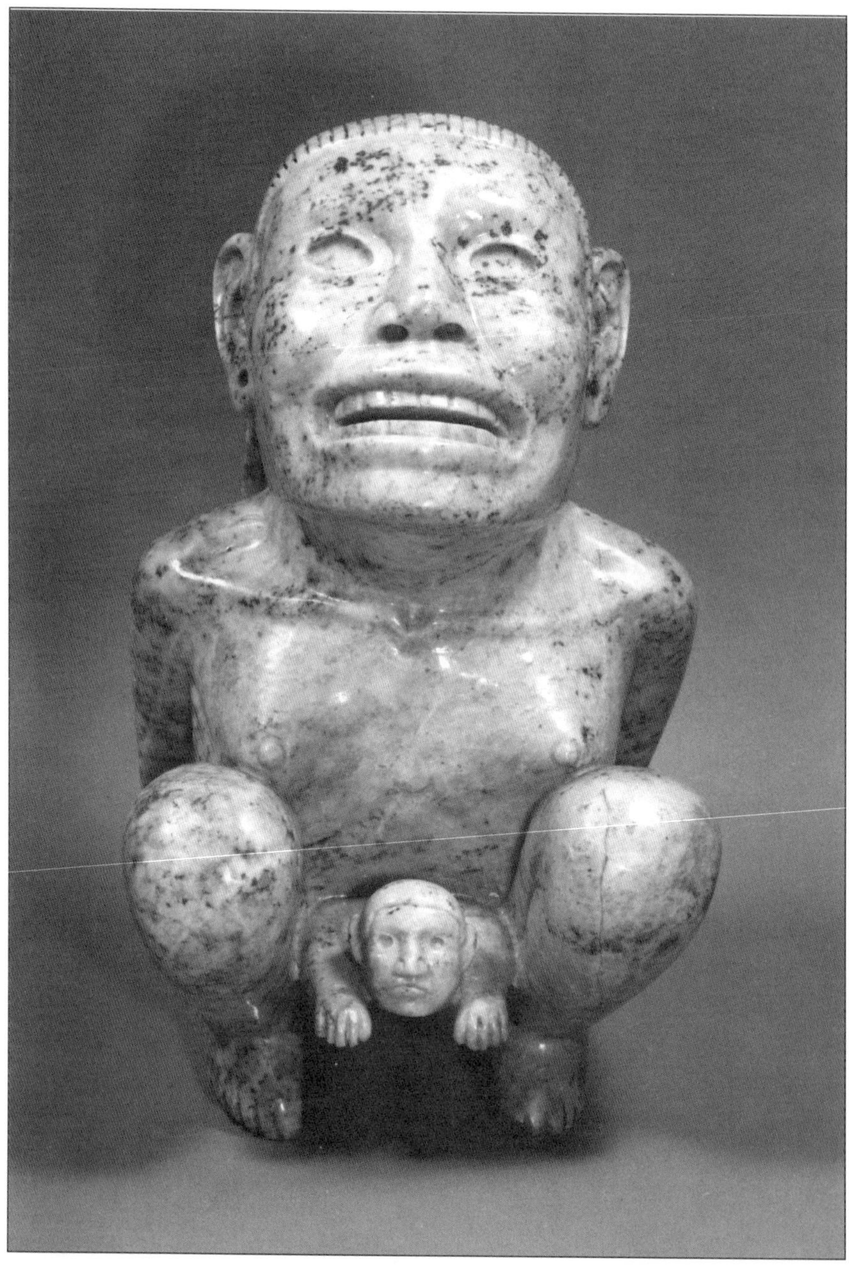

Tlazolteotl, the Goddess of Childbirth. Dumbarton Oaks Research Library and Collections, Washington, D.C.

the child is, first, when its head presents with the hands bent upon the thighs, and having its head directly applied to the mouth of the womb; and next to that, when it descends by the feet, and there is no turning aside. All the other positions except these are preternatural. Or from the secundines, either because the membranes cannot be torn, owing to their thickness; or because they have been torn prematurely, owing to their thinness; for when the waters are evacuated unseasonably, the foetus gets out with difficulty, from the dryness of the parts. From external circumstances, either from cold contracting or immoderate heat dissipating the powers, or from some accidental occurrence. Wherefore, if the difficulty of parturition arise from constriction, and, as it were, impaction of the foetus, we must first endeavor to produce relaxation by injecting frequently hot sweet-oil with the decoction of fenugreek, or mallows, of linseed, or with eggs as a pareogoric. Then we must apply cataplasms to the pubes, abdomen, and loins, or linseed or of honied water, or of oil and water; and use hipbaths of a similar nature. We must also avail ourselves of the relaxation produced by baths, if neither fever nor any other cause prohibit; and the woman is to be moved on a couch in a moderately warm air. Some have had recourse to powerful shaking, and have applied sternutatories. If the woman be in low spirits, she is to be encouraged; and if she is inexperienced in labour, she is to be directed to keep in her breath strongly, and to press down to the flanks. If she be in a swoon, she is to be resuscitated by such strong-smelling things as are not stimulant; and when moderately recovered, she is to be supported with a little food. A woman that is fat is to be placed in bed in a prone position, bending her knees upon her thighs, in order that the womb, being carried to the abdomen, may present with its mouth direct. By means of the fingers the mouth is to be smeared with cerates or fatty substances, and gently dilated. And if there be any complaint in the parts, it must be previously attended to; and hardened faeces when retained must be expelled by an emollient clyster. The membranes may be divided either by the fingers or by a scalpel concealed within them, the left hand directing it. And some of the fatty liquids may be thrown up into the uterus by a syringe. When the foetus is in preternatural position, we may restore the natural position by sometimes pressing it back, sometimes drawing it down, sometimes pushing it aside and sometimes rectifying the whole. If a hand or foot protrude, we must not seize upon the limb and drag it down, for thereby it will be the more wedged in or may be dislocated or fractured; but fixing the fingers about the shoulders or hip joint of the foetus, the part that had protruded is to be restored to its proper position. If there be a wrong position of the whole foetus, attended with impaction, we must first push it upwards from the mouth of the womb, than lay hold of it, and direct it properly to the mouth of the uterus. If more than one child have descended, they are to be raised upwards again, and then brought downwards. Everything is to be done gently, and without pressure, the parts being smeared with oil. The time for placing the woman on the stool is when the mouth of the womb is open and meets the finger, and when rupture of the membranes is at hand. If, owing to the death of the child, or any other cause, it do not advance, we must proceed to embryotomy.

Appendix II

From *The Anatomy of Melancholy*

Robert Burton (1577–1640 C.E.)

Because Lodovicus Mercatus . . . and Rodericus a Castro . . . with others have vouchsafed, in their works not long since published, to write two just treatises *de Melancholia Virginum, Monialium, et Viduarum* [virgins', nuns', and widows' melancholy] as a peculiar species of Melancholy distinct from the rest (for it much differs from that which commonly befalls men and other women, as having only one cause proper to women alone), I may not omit, in this general survey of melancholy symptoms, to set down the particular signs of such parties so misaffected.

"The causes are assigned out of Hippocrates, Cleopatra, Moschion, and those old *gynaeciorum scriptores,* of this feral malady, in more ancient Maids, Widows and barren Women, *ob septum transversum violatum,* saith Mercatus, by reason of the midriff or *diaphragma,* heart and brain offended with those vicious vapours which come from menstrous blood; *inflammationem arteriae circa dorsum,* Rodericus adds, an inflammation of the back, which with the rest if offended by that fuliginous exhalation of corrupt seed, troubling the brain, heart, and mind; the brain I say, not in essence, but by consent, *universa enim hujus affectus causa ab utero pendet, et a sanguinis menstrui malitia,* for, in a word, the whole malady proceeds from that inflammation, putridity, black smoky vapours and from thence comes care, sorrow, and anxiety, obfuscation of spirits, agony, desperation, and the like, which are intended or remitted, from any amatory propensity or any other violent object or perturbation of mind. This melancholy may happen to Widows, with much care and sorrow, as frequently it doth, by reason of a sudden alteration of their accustomed course of life. To such as lie in childbed, *ob suppressam purgationem*; but to Nuns and more ancient Maids, and some barren Women, for the causes above said, 'tis more familiar, it happens to these more frequently than to the rest. The several cures of this infirmity, concerning diet, which must be very sparing, phlebotomy, physick, internal, external remedies, are at large in great variety . . . but the best and surest remedy of all is to see them well placed and married to good husbands in due time. How odious and abominable are those superstitions and rash vows . . . so as to bind and enforce men and women to vow virginity, to lead a single life against the laws of nature . . . to suppress the vigor of youth. . . . It troubles me to think of, much more to relate, those frequent aborts and murdering of infants in their Nunneries, their notorious fornications . . . those rapes, incests, and adulteries.

APPENDIX III

The Pill

By 1970, manufacturers competed heavily with various mixes of estrogen and progesterone. The dosage had to prevent pregnancy but not promote pathological changes. Consequently, a plethora of pills was manufactured. Those listed below are available in the United States and the United Kingdom.

C-QUENS	.08 mg mestanol/2 mg chlormadinone
ENOVID 5 mg	.075 mg mestranol/5 mg norethynodrel
ENOVID-E	.1 mg mestranol/2. 5 mg norethynodrel
NORINYL 2 mg	.1 mg mestranol/2 mg norethynodrel
NORINYL 10 mg	.06 mg mestranol/10 mg norethindrone
NORINYL-1 20 day	.05 mg mestranol/1 mg norethindrone
NORINYL-1 21 day	.05 mg mestranol/1 mg norethindrone
NORINYL-1 28 day	.05 mg mestranol/1 mg norethindrone
NORINYL 1+80 1 day	.08 mg mestranol 1 mg norethindrone
NORINYL 1+80 28 day	.08 mg mestanol/1 mg norethindrone

NORLESTRIN 1 mg	.05 mg ethinyl estradiol/1 mg norethindrone
NORLESTRIN 1 mg 21 day	.05 mg ethinyl estradiol/1 mg norethindrone
NORLESTRIN 1 mg 28 day	.05 mg ethinyl estradiol/1 mg norethindrone
NORLESTRIN Fe 1 mg	.05 mg ethinyl estradiol/1 mg norethindrone and ferrous fumarate
NORQUEN	.08 mg mestranol/2 mg norethindrone
ORACON	.1 mg ethinyl estradiol/25 dimethisterone
ORTHO-NOVUM 1+80 21 day	.08 mg mestranol/1 mg norethindrone
ORTHO-NOVUM 1+80 28 day	.08 mg mestranol/1 mg norethindrone
ORTHO-NOVUM mg	.05 mg mestranol/1 mg norethindrone
ORTHO-NOVUM 1 mg 28 day	.05 mg mestranol/1 mg norethindrone
ORTHO-NOVUM 2 mg	.1 mg mestranol/2 mg norethindrone
ORTHO-NOVUM 10 mg	.06 mg mestranol/10 mg norethindrone
ORTHO-NOVUM 2 mg	.08 mg mestranol/2 mg norethindrone
OVRAL	.05 mg ethinyl estradiol/.5 mg norgestrel
OVULEN	1 mg mestranol/1 mg ethynodiol diacetate
OVULEN-21	1 mg mestranol/1 mg ethynodiol diacetate
OVULEN-28	.1 mg mestanol/1 mg ethynodiol diacetate
PROVEST	0.5 mg ethinyl estradiol/10 mg medroxyprogesterone

APPENDIX IV

The "Birthezz" Correspondence

Dear Ms. Thompson,

Please forgive me for not replying sooner to your letter about "Birthezz."

I was a resident at the Queen Victoria Hospital in Johannesburg when Professor Heyns, who was my chief, was doing research on what we called "The Birth Suit." My wife was pregnant with our second child and she used the Birth Suit, which was used for abdominal decompression. The idea was that by using abdominal decompression you increased blood flow to the uterus as well as to the placenta. The increased blood flow would hopefully improve placental profusion and as a consequence you would have more intelligent babies as well as decreasing the incidence of pre-eclamptic toxemia.

Unfortunately, in those days, we did not have the apparatus to measure increased blood flow or increased profusion of the placenta. The testing of the babies was also somewhat crude and not very reliable.

I do not have a picture of the suit. The suit was made out of plastic with a zipper all the way from the toes to the top of the suit, which was level with the clavicle and fitted under the arms. There was a fiberglass dome which fitted over the patient's abdomen and slotted into a back rest made out of fiberglass which supported the back. The patient sat in a type of lounge chair. The decompression was obtained by connecting the dome to a regular vacuum cleaner. There was a second valve which the patient closed manually and so a vacuum was produced to decompress the suit. The patient would decompress for a minute, release compression for 30 seconds, and repeat the procedure over a 20-minute period for three times a week from mid–second trimester.

The decompression suit was used for almost three years in South Africa and was never available commercially. I am not sure but I think that Professor Justus Hofmeyr of the Department of Obstetrics and Gynecology, University of Witwatersrand Medical, was considering doing some research work on the decompression suit. Professor Heyns has long since passed away. The technician who helped design the apparatus, Jack Graham, has also passed away.

I hope this note will be of some value to you. Should you want to call me or fax me, I will try to answer any other questions.

Please feel free to contact me.

Best regards,

Mervyn Hurwitz

Bibliography

Allport, Gordon W. *The Nature of Prejudice.* Garden City: Doubleday Anchor Books, 1958.

Anonymous. "Impairment of the Voice in Female Singers." *Journal of the American Medical Association,* Vol. 268, No. 2, 1992.

Augustine. *Confessions* (translated by Henry Chadwick). Oxford: Oxford University Press, 1991.

Barstow, Anne Llewellyn. *Witchcraze: A New History of the European Witch Hunts.* New York: Pandora, 1994.

Bettmann, Otto L. *The Pictorial History of Medicine.* Baltimore: Charles C. Thomas, 1957.

Boston Women's Health Collective, The. *The New Our Bodies, Ourselves.* New York: Touchstone, 1984.

Boyar, Paul, and Stephen Nissenbaum. *Salem Possessed: The Social Origins of Witchcraft.* Cambridge: Harvard University Press, 1974.

Brace, Richard. *The Making of the Modern World: From the Renaissance to the Present.* New York: Holt-Reinhard, 1960.

Brauner, Sigrid. *Fearless Wives and Frightened Shrews.* Amherst: University of Massachusetts Press, 1992.

Bullough, Vern L. *Sex, Society and History.* New York: Science History Publications, 1976.

Bullough, Vern L., and James Brundage. *Sexual Practices in the Medieval Church.* Amherst, N.Y.: Prometheus Books, 1995.

Bullough, Vern L., and Bonnie Bullough. *Sexual Attitudes: Myths and Realities.* Amherst, N.Y.: Prometheus Books, 1995.

Bullough, Vern L., and Bonnie Bullough. *The Subordinate Sex: A History of Attitudes Toward Women.* Urbana: University of Illinois Press, 1973.

Bullough, Vern L., Brenda Shelton, and Sarah Slavin. *The Subordinated Sex: A History of Attitudes Toward Women.* Athens: University of Georgia Press, 1988.

Burgan, Mary. *Illness, Gender and Writing.* Baltimore: Johns Hopkins University Press, 1994.

Burton, Robert. *The Anatomy of Melancholy, Volume 1* (edited by the Reverend A.R. Shilleto, M.A.; reprinted from the 1893 edition, London: George Bell & Sons). New York: AMS Press, 1973.

Chesler, Ellen. *Woman of Valor: Margaret Sanger and the Birth Control Movement in America.* New York: Doubleday, 1992.

Clark, Margaret. "Medical Anthropology and the Redefining of Human Nature." *Human Organization,* Vol. 52, No. 3, 1993.

Clendening, Logan, ed. *Source Book of Medical History* (reprint of the 1942 edition). New York: Dover Publications, 1960.

Corea, Gina. *The Hidden Malpractice: How American Medicine Treats Women as Patients and Professionals.* New York: William Morrow and Company, Inc., 1977

Curran, William J. "Court Ordered Caesarean Sections Received Judicial Defeat." *New England Journal of Medicine,* Vol. 323, No. 7, 1990.

Dally, Ann. *Women under the Knife.* New York: Routledge, 1992.

Davis-Floyd, Robbie E. *Birth as an American Rite of Passage.* Berkeley: University of California Press, 1992.

Demos, John Putnam. *Entertaining Satan.* New York: Oxford University Press, 1982.

Dictionary of Scientific Biography. New York: Charles Scribner's Sons, 1970.

Dixon, Laurinda. *Perilous Chastity*. Ithaca: Cornell University Press, 1995.

Donegan, Jane. *Women and Men Midwives*. Westport: Greenwood Press, 1978.

Donnison, Jean. *Midwives and Medical Men*. London: Heinemann, 1977.

Duby, Georges, and Michelle Perrot, eds. *A History of Women in the West, Volume 1: From Ancient Goddesses to Christian Saints*. Cambridge: Belknap Press, 1992.

———. *A History of Women in the West, Volume 2: Silences of the Middles Ages*. Cambridge: Belknap Press, 1992.

———. *A History of Women in the West, Volume 3: Renaissance and Enlightenment Paradoxes*. Cambridge: Belknap Press, 1993.

Eco, Umberto. *The Name of the Rose*. New York: Warner Books, 1984.

Ehrenreich, Barbara, and Deirdre English. *For Her Own Good: 150 Years of the Experts' Advice to Women*. New York: Anchor Books, 1978.

———. *Complaints and Disorders: The Sexual Politics of Sickness*. New York: The Feminist Press, 1973.

———. *Witches, Midwives and Nurses: A History of Women Healers*. New York: The Feminist Press, 1973.

Fielding, Garrison H. *An Introduction to the History of Medicine*. Philadelphia: W.B. Saunders Company, 1929.

Foos, Laurie. *Ex Utero*. Minneapolis: Coffee House Press, 1996.

Fox, Sally. *The Medieval Woman: An Illuminated Book of Days*. New York: Little, Brown, 1985.

Francoeur, Robert. *Utopian Motherhood: New Trends in Human Reproduction*. New York: Doubleday, 1970.

Geller, Jeffrey L., and Maxine Harris. *Women of the Asylum*. New York: Anchor Books, 1994.

Goodman, Louis S., and Alfred Gilman. *Pharmacological Basis of Therapeutics* (seventh edition). New York: Macmillan, 1985.

Grun, Bernard. *The Timetables of History*. New York: Simon & Schuster, 1991.

Harding, Sandra, and Jean F. O'Barr. *Sex and Scientific Inquiry.* Chicago: University of Chicago Press, 1987.

Harksen, Sibylle. *Women of the Middle Ages.* New York: Abner Schram/Universe Books, 1975.

Hollick, F. *The Origin of Life and Process of Reproduction in Plants and Animals, with the Anatomy and Physiology of the Human Generative System, Male and Female, and the Causes, Prevention and Cure of the Special Disease to which It Is Liable. A Plain, Practical Treatise for Popular Use.* Philadelphia: David McKay, 1902.

Holme, Thea. *Prinny's Daughter.* London: Hamish Hamilton, 1976.

Holy Bible (Pilgrim Edition). New York: Oxford University Press, 1952.

Jefferis, B.G., and J.L. Nichols. *Safe Counsel, or Practical Eugenics.* New York: Intext Press, 1928.

Jones, Howard W., and Georgeanna Seegar Jones. *Novak's Textbook of Gynecology* (tenth edition). Baltimore: Williams & Wilkins, 1981.

Jones, Vivien, ed. *Women in the Eighteenth Century.* London: Routledge, 1990.

Karlen, Arno. *Sexuality and Homosexuality: A New View.* New York: W.W. Norton & Co., 1971.

Karlsen, Carol F. *The Devil in the Shape of a Woman.* New York: W.W. Norton & Co., 1987.

Kay, Thomas. "A Study of Sterility, Its Causes and Treatments." *Journal of the American Medical Association,* Vol. 265, No. 6, 1991.

Kennedy, Brian P., and Davis Coakley, eds. *The Anatomy Lesson.* Dublin: National Gallery of Ireland, 1992.

King, Margaret. *Women of the Renaissance.* Chicago: University of Chicago Press, 1991.

Klein, H. Arthur. *Graphic Worlds of Peter Bruegel the Elder.* New York: Dover Publications, 1963.

Kuhn, Thomas. *The Structure of Scientific Revolutions* (second edition). Chicago: University of Chicago Press, 1967.

Leavitt, Judith Walzer. *Brought to Bed.* New York: Oxford University Press, 1986.

———, ed. *Women and Health in America.* Madison: University of Wisconsin Press, 1984.

Legato, Marianne J. "Tomorrow the World." *The Female Patient,* Vol. 21, No. 4, 1996.

Lifton, Robert Jay. *The Nazi Doctors: Medical Killing and the Psychology of Genocide.* New York: Basic Books, 1986.

Lind, L.R. *Pre-Vesalian Anatomy: Biography, Translations, Documents.* Philadelphia: The American Philosophical Society, 1975.

Lyons, Albert, and R. Joseph Petrucelli. *Medicine: An Illustrated History.* New York: Harry N. Abrams, 1987.

Maccurdy, Edward, ed. *The Notebooks of Leonardo da Vinci.* New York: George Braziller, 1956.

Macdonald, Michael. *Witchcraft and Hysteria in Elizabethan London: Edward Jorden and the Mary Glover Case.* New York: Tavistock/Routledge, 1991.

Magner, Lois. *A History of Medicine.* New York: Marcel Dekker, Inc., 1992.

McGregor, Deborah Kuhn. *Sexual Surgey and the Origins of Gynecology.* New York: Garland, 1989.

Mills, Jane. *Womanwords: A Dictionary of Words About Women.* New York: Henry Holt, 1989.

Minkowski, William. "Women Healers in the Middle Ages: Selected Aspects of their History." *American Journal of Public Health,* Vol. 82, No. 2, 1992.

Monter, E. William. "Witchcraft." *Grolier MultiMedia Encyclopedia,* Version 7.0, 1995.

O'Malley, Charles D. *Andreas Vesalius of Brussels.* Berkeley: University of California Press, 1965.

Ranke-Heinemann, Uta. *Eunuchs for the Kingdom of Heaven: Women, Sexuality and the Catholic Church.* New York: Penguin, 1990.

Rohe, George. "Lactational Insanity." *Journal of the American Medical Association,* Vol. 270, No. 10, 1993.

Rosen, Barbara. *Witchcraft.* New York: Taplinger Publishing Co., 1972.

Rothman, David, Steven Marcus, and Stephanie Kiceluk, eds. *Medicine and Western Civilization.* New Brunswick: Rutgers University Press, 1995.

Russell, Jeffrey Burton. *Witchcraft in the Middle Ages.* Ithaca: Cornell University Press, 1972.

Sanday, Peggy. *Female Power and Male Dominance: The Origins of Sexual Inequality.* New York: Cambridge University Press, 1981.

Saunders, J. B. deC. M., and Charles D. O'Malley. *The Illustrations from the Works of Andreas Vesalius.* New York: Dover Publications, 1973.

Sawday, Jonathan. *The Body Emblazoned.* London: Routledge, 1995.

Schleiner, Winfried. *Medical Ethics in the Renaissance.* Washington, D.C.: Georgetown University Press, 1995.

Seldes, George. *The Great Quotations.* New York: Carol Publishing Group, 1993.

Shorter, Edward. *A History of Women's Bodies.* New York: Basic Books, 1982.

Sigerist, Henry. *Civilization and Disease.* Chicago: University of Chicago Press, 1970.

Singer, Charles. *A Short History of Anatomy from the Greeks to Harvey.* New York: Dover Publications, 1957.

Sisson, Septimus, and James Daniel Grossman. *The Anatomy of Domestic Animals.* Philadelphia: W.B. Saunders Company, 1938.

Slavney, Phillip. *Perspectives on Hysteria.* Baltimore: Johns Hopkins University Press, 1990.

Spencer, Robert, et al. *The Native Americans: Ethnology and Backgrounds of the North American Indians.* New York: Harper and Row, 1977.

Stage, Sarah. *Female Complaints: Lydia Pinkham and the Business of Women's Medicine.* New York: W.W. Norton & Co., 1979.

Straus, Walter L., ed. *The Complete Engravings, Etchings, and Drypoints of Albrecht Dürer.* New York: Dover Publications, 1973.

Szasz, Thomas. *The Manufacture of Madness.* New York: Harper and Row, 1986.

Thompson, Morton. *The Cry and the Covenant.* Garden City: Doubleday, 1949.

Thoms, Herbert. *Classical Contributions to Obstetrics and Gynecology.* Springfield: Charles C. Thomas, 1935.

Ussher, Jane M. *Women's Madness: Misogyny or Mental Illness.* Amherst: University of Massachusetts Press, 1991.

Veith, Ilza. *Hysteria: The History of a Disease.* Chicago: University of Chicago Press, 1965.

Walker, Barbara G. *The Women's Encyclopedia of Myths and Secrets.* Edison: Castle Books, 1996.

Wallace, Robert. *The World of Leonardo.* New York: Time Inc., 1966.

Weideger, Paula. *History's Mistress.* London: Penguin, 1986.

———. *Menstruation and Menopause: The Physiology and Psychology, the Myth and the Reality.* New York: Alfred A. Knopf, 1976.

Weigel, Gustave, and McNaspy, C.J. "Catholic Church: Doctrine." *The Encyclopedia Americana International Edition, Volume 6.* New York: Americana Corporation, 1971.

Wertz, Richard W., and Dorothy C. Wertz. *Lying In: A History of Childbirth in America.* New Haven: Yale University Press, 1977.

Willy, A., L. Vander, O. Fisher, et al. *The Illustrated Encyclopedia of Sex.* Royton Publishing Co., 1977.

Wynn, Ralph M. *Biology of the Uterus.* New York: Plenum Press, 1977.

Zigroser, Carl. *Medicine and the Artist.* New York: Dover Publications, 1970.

Index